T.E. HALL: Technique and Diagnosis

Edited and compiled by
Russell John White

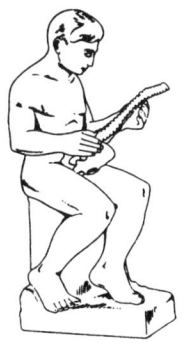

Institute of Classical Osteopathy

Published by: The Institute of Classical Osteopathy
The Unicorn Centre
Tanner's Yard
Shrewsbury
Shropshire
SY1 1XB

Copyright: Russell John White and
The Institute of Classical Osteopathy

This is a limited edition of 500 copies

COPY No. *111*

All rights reserved. No part of this publication may by reproduced, stored in a retrieval system, or transmitted, in any form or by any means, electronic, photocopying, recording or otherwise without the prior permission in writing of the Copyright holders.

ISBN Number 0 9530294 0 9

Produced in Great Britain by
Rea Valley Printers Limited
The Old Bakery
Pontesbury
Shropshire
SY5 0PY

ACKNOWLEDGEMENTS

Thanks to: John Wernham for his inspiration and example.

Dr C. Dutton (Honorary Senior Clinical Lecturer at the London College of Osteopathic Medicine) who kindly loaned his unique photo album of Hall demonstrating technique, which provided the photographs for this book.

Mr C. Campbell for his help and encouragement.

Susan and Karen for their patience and practical help.

Contents

Physiological Movements of the Spine	9
Mechanics of Lesion Diagnosis in the Pelvis	27
Diagnosis and Treatment of Psoas Muscle Conditions	40
Diagnosis and Treatment of the Low Back	51
Two Man Technique	59
Diagnosis and Treatment of the Lower Dorsal Spine *(with P.A. Jackson)*	65
The Occipito-Atlantal Articulation	72
The Elbow	82
The Shoulder	90
The Knee	104
The Foot	113

PREFACE

T.E. Hall was regarded by his contemporaries as being the most accomplished osteopathic technician of his time. Nothing is known of his early history, except that he joined the army and became a musician. He later joined the Debroy Somers band, and we find him on board ship as a member of the orchestra, and suffering from the effects of a chronic knee injury, a legacy from the football field. Among the passengers there was an elderly American osteopath, and the knee and the musician were dramatically relieved. The year was 1925 and on returning to London, Hall registered as a student with J.M. Littlejohn, at his address in Dover Street.

As he approached seniority during his student years, his natural gift in the field of osteopathic technique began to emerge, and to lay the foundations of a long, and fruitful career under the guiding hand of J.M. Littlejohn. After the early days in Vincent Square, the British School of Osteopathy occupied temporary accommodation at Abbey House in nearby Victoria Street, before becoming permanently established at 16 Buckingham Gate in 1930. Having graduated in 1929, Hall joined the faculty of the School, teaching osteopathic technique, a subject in which he excelled, and taking the office of Vice-Dean in 1934.

It was during these formative years in the life of the School that he visited American colleges, and a life-long friendship with Harrison H. Fryette was formed.

It was his unswerving loyalty during the difficult years following the failure of the Parliamentary Bill in 1935 and, more particularly, during the war years, that prevented final disaster from overtaking the only school of osteopathy in Great Britain at that time. It has been said that "but for Hall the School would not have survived the war".

In the 1950's new influences began to deviate from the principles laid down by J.M. Littlejohn, and promulgated by Hall. It was at this time that the Osteopathic Institute of Applied Technique (now know as the Institute of Classical Osteopathy) was formed. Hall made the original suggestion that such an organisation should be formed and became one of the founder-members. He taught, and demonstrated, his techniques to the membership and these have been preserved in recordings, on film and in the Year Books published by the Institute.

Hall was not a prolific writer. Nearly all of the articles in this book are based on lectures and demonstrations given by him in the late 1950's and 60's. He was an entertaining and knowledgeable speaker, although somewhat prone to straying from the subject. Many of his anecdotes and asides have been included in the articles and they help to give a hint of his unique style of presentation.

His association with Fryette further refined his already high degree of diagnostic and technical ability. He had no time for what he called "crack merchants" and, according to John Wernham "when demonstrating to students he would often manipulate the model's neck until all the cracks had been taken out of it and only then tell the student to get on with the adjustment."

For Hall, the art of osteopathy demanded a thorough knowledge of the physiological movements of the spine, a high degree of diagnostic and palpatory skills and the technical ability to deal with the underlying conditions. What would he have made of the comments by a recent graduate of the B.S.O. that they "do not do manipulation because it is too difficult"?

The Institute of Classical Osteopathy exists to help stem the general decline in standards of manipulative and diagnostic skills and continues the work of its founders Hall, Wernham, Proby, Jackson and others.

After a long and distinguished career T.E. Hall died on the 24th March 1979. We shall not see his like again.

R.J. White
Asterley Hall
Asterley

For those interested in finding out more about the technique and diagnostic skills of T.E. Hall, the Institute of Classical Osteopathy has produced a video of his work. We are fortunate that mainly due to the dedication and the foresight of John Wernham, a considerable amount of 35mm footage of Hall in action has survived. This has been edited and transcribed onto video tape under the supervision of Mr C. Campbell, Principal of the Irish College of Classical Osteopathy. Copies can be obtained from the Institute of Classical Osteopathy. Recordings of some of his original lectures are also available.

PHYSIOLOGICAL MOVEMENTS OF THE SPINE

As the subject matter of this paper provides the basis of all scientific spinal technique, I ask your indulgence while I quote rather extensively from a lecture given at the annual convention of the American Osteopathic Association, in 1936, by Dr H.H. Fryette, on *'Technique and Nomenclature'*. (1) Dr Fryette says, "as a profession, if we were to take stock of ourselves, we should be most proud of our technique. Our individual success and the success of our science depends upon our skill to apply our knowledge, but as a matter of fact, while each individual thinks his technique is scientific, most are quite willing to confess that the technique of the profession as a whole is very mediocre." We all get good results, but is that due to the wonderful principles of osteopathy and the ability of the body to cure itself, or to our unusual ability to apply those osteopathic principles?"

Our profession is young, and we have had so many new ideas to develop and co-ordinate with our practice, that we may be pardoned if we find ourselves in more or less of a fog, but I cannot help but feel that we have been very negligent in developing our technique.

The colleges should have a Technique Association made up of all the teachers of technique and the outstanding technicians of the profession, and it is my hope that eventually this Osteopathic Institute of Applied Technique will serve a similar purpose to the profession in this country.

As every professor of technique knows, the subject is extremely hard to teach, not only because it it is difficult to get a student to visualise the lesion, but harder still for him to learn to palpate it. Therefore, it has been my thought that if we could adopt a terminology that is descriptive of the lesion, it is not only easier to diagnose but easier to adjust.

Most spinal lesions have resulted from the faulty reception of force, from motion; therefore, it is very illuminating, in view of the fact that we anticipate ultimate correction, to know as nearly as possible through what series of motions the vertebrae moved when the lesion was produced in order that we may reverse these movements in the correction. Simply to say that a vertebra is extended, flexed, or rotated, and to name all lesions in all three sections of the spine as such, seems to me to indicate a complete lack of understanding of the physiological movements of the spine.

It is theoretically possible to have a spinal lesion in the position of bi-lateral flexion or extension, although it seldom happens, but it is impossible to have a vertebra rotated unless it is in the position of extension, rotation sidebending or flexion sidebending rotation. To say that a vertebra is rotated (with the complement of lateral flexion) means absolutely nothing from the stand-point of diagnosis or correction.

FLEXION AND EXTENSION

In any new science it becomes necessary at times to coin new words or adopt old phrases to new meanings:

Flexion means to bend.

Extension means to straighten

If one was speaking of the torso in relation to the lower limbs, flexion would naturally mean forward bending, and extension would mean bringing the trunk back in line with the legs, and over-extension would mean to bend the body back off perpendicular.

These terms have always been used in anatomy to mean just that, but when it comes to osteopathic technique it is an entirely different matter, for here we are speaking of the spine with its ventral and dorsal curves.

When we bend the trunk forward we extend the lumbar and cervical ventral curves, and we increase the dorsal curve. Also, when we bend the trunk backwards we increase the lumbar and cervical ventral curves and extend the dorsal curve. Therefore, in speaking of the movement of the different areas of the spine, if we wish to use the terms Flexion and Extension, it is necessary to apply the terms to each area of the spine specifically and not the spine as a whole. This becomes more obvious when one observes the behaviour of the different areas of the spine when it is side bent from the position of flexion or extension, or when the spine is in neutral.

For, when any given area of the spine is in neutral and is side bent, the bodies rotate to the convexity and the movements occur in the sequence of side bending rotation, but if any given area of the spine is in extension or extreme flexion, the bodies rotate to the concavity when the spine is side bent in the sequence of rotation side bending.

It becomes quite obvious, therefore, that if one is to recognise the physiological movements of the spine at all, that the terms Flexion and Extension must be used in relation to the various areas of the spine and not to the spine as a whole.

I would suggest that the vertebral lesion should be designated by the position in which it is; for example, as a flexion, side bending rotation lesion of, say, the fourth dorsal, or as an extension, rotation-side-bending lesion of the fifth lumbar.

This terminology will apply to 99% of the spinal lesions. There are straight impaction lesions, and one may find irregular lesions caused from a direct blow or a chiropractic treatment. These irregular lesions must be defined as they are found.

This particular terminology is especially helpful in building a corrective technique, for all that is necessary in correction is to reverse the sequence of movements that produce the lesion.

This sounds so familiar to us today and so academically scientific that we take it for granted. But it was not always so. When Dr Fryette introduced these physiological movements of the spine to the profession, he was following research begun on the same lines by (2) Dr R.W. Lovett, an M.D. of Boston, U.S.A., who announced his conclusions in his book which was published in 1907 under the title of *'Lateral Curvature of the Spine and Round Shoulders'*. He, Dr Lovett, undoubtedly undertook this research in order to learn more of the etiology of spinal curvature, knowing nothing and not even suspecting the existence of the individual osteopathic "Still" lesion we are so familiar with today. Had he done so I am sure some of his conclusions would have been different, but his book shows he was only concerned with gross structural curvatures and their treatment. On his conclusions (3) Dr Fryette in the manuscript of his new book on *'Applied Osteopathy'*, just published, has this to say:

> "Dr Lovett observed that there were two dominant factors that control, or at least modify, the mechanical behaviour of the spine. They are the articulating facets and the bodies of the vertebrae. Dr Lovett sawed the spine down through the pedicles. He then had the anterior part of the spine, the bodies and the intervertebral discs in one column and the posterior part of the spine, the facets, in the other column".

In experimenting with these two columns, Dr Lovett observed that when the column of bodies was side-bent, under load it tended to collapse toward the convexity, as a pile of blocks would do. Whereas, the column of facets behaved like a flexible ruler or a blade of grass, it was necessary to rotate it before it could be side-bent. Therefore, it is obvious that in the intact spine, to the degree that the facets are in control, they direct and govern rotation.

Notwithstanding these facts, Dr Lovett's conclusions in regard to rotation in the various areas of the spine are as follows:

(1) In the Lumbar. "The rotation accompanying sidebending in the lumbar is *always* in the bodies turning to the concavity of the lateral curve."

(2) In the Dorsal Region. "The rotation of the vertebrae in sidebending in the dorsal region is always toward the convexity of the lateral curve."

(3) In the Cervical Region. In the cervical region, "sidebending is accompanied by rotation of the bodies of the vertebrae to the concavity of the lateral curve, as in the Lumbar."

Dr Fryette adds:

> "These statements are true for the various areas of the spine positioned as they were when Dr Lovett performed his experiments, but they are not true in the lumbar when that area is in neutral or moderate flexion. Or

in the dorsal when it is side-bent from the position of moderate extension."

This, then, was the accepted position up to the time when Dr Fryette gave his celebrated paper to the American Osteopathic Association in 1918 and of which he says quite simply:

"I was naive enough to think that the profession would accept my work at once and with enthusiasm but this was not the case."

Indeed, it was not, and the physiological movements of the spine as such were, I am sorry to say, left severely alone for many years by the profession, who did not realise that a great and profound discovery was being lost to osteopathy until early in the 1930's, since when hardly an article has been written or a lecture given on technique without extensive reference to these movements. I think it is only fair to state that our late Dean (4) Dr J. Martin Littlejohn, never ceased teaching this subject, and what I am trying to pass on today is the result of his teaching in 1926, 1927 and 1928 when I was a student at the British School of Osteopathy, first in Vincent Square and later in Abbey House. In fact, all the original research into these physiological movements was carried out by Dr Fryette while he was the professor of technique at the Littlejohn College of Osteopathy in Chicago – this college being founded by the late Dr Martin Littlejohn and his two brothers, in 1900. However, to proceed, all authorities today are agreed on the fact that the dominating factor controlling the physiological movements of the spine are:

(i) the bodies of the vertebrae and intervertebral discs, and

(ii) the articulating facets, ligaments and cartilages.

There is, however, a slight difference of opinion on the terminolgy to be used to describe these movements, or rather the interpretation of the nomenclature.

Some speak of flexion and extension of the spine as applied to the forward and backward bending of the trunk on the thighs, while others prefer to accept flexion and extension as applied to the separate curves or areas of the spine. With only one or two exceptions, current literature reveals that the majority accept the latter viewpoint and I personally do so, too. It is known to us all that the mechanics of the spine are evolved round three physiological curves, extending from the axis to the lumbo-sacral articulation, and are named the lumbar, cervical and dorsal curves. I stress the axis to lumbo-sacral because in pure mechanics of the spine the occipital atlantal articulation and the articulation of the sacrum with the two iliacs reverse the mechanics of the movement in relation to the rest of the spine.

At the same time the pelvis, with its sacral curve must be considered as one of the primary posterior curves which can and often does greatly influence the development of the physiological movements of the rest of the spine.

In this respect I would like to say a few words on the origin and the development of the spinal curves, both posterior and anterior.

(5) Just for a few minutes, let us pause and reflect on this marvellous mechanical structure which is the body. This reflection tells us that the body is an animated structure, animated by its own vital activity – it manufactures its own motive power, it also controls, regulates and maintains the supply of these vital forces necessary to motivity and animation. In fact, so intimately are the two bound together that if the motive power fails animation fails and with animation gone, life is gone and the structures become subject to the laws of gravity and fails also; it is as simple as that. The same is true in reverse.

We know that this living vital force which animates the structure is represented by the physiological function of the body and we therefore can only interpret this to mean that the foundations of body mechanics, while resting on the physical principles of pure mechanics, must take account of the fact that the skeletal structures and their adaptive functions are modified and, to a great extent, brought under the influence of the responsive action of muscles, etc., under the stimulus of nerve action.

This means, therefore, that in the application of the laws of physics to the mechanism of the human body, in oppositon to the laws and force of gravity, we must, of necessity, study not physics alone, but physics in relation to physiology and attempt to combine both. This is why Dr Littlejohn explained the physiological movements of the spine as a study in physiological physics.

To do this thoroughly, of course, it would be necessary to revert to the body in Utero and follow developments from there, but to cover this subject – 'The Embryology of Physiology' – is essentially someone else's province, so, for our purpose, I shall only give a very brief resumé.

As we all know, before the outlines of the foetus are developed, the cells which form the mass which is to be the embryo become differentiated into three embryological types of tissue.

These are:
(1) THE ECTODERM which, generally speaking, gives rise to the central and peripheral Nervous System.
(2) THE ENTODERM which gives rise mainly to the Enteral System, and
(3) THE MESODERM from which is derived the eventual skeletal and muscular systems and which is divided into the mesodermic somites. The sclerotomic parts of two somites representing one vertebra in the future segmentation of the spinal column. Within three to five weeks, these germinal layers commence division with the Medullary Groove from the Mid-Dorsal region and continue

development until:
through the ECTODERM, the Nervous System commences to grow;
through the ENTODERM, the organs begin to take definite shape;
through the MESODERM AND MESODERMIC SOMITES, the future skeletal musculature commences development and the spine begins to take on a definite order of segmentation and follows the development of the Nervous and Enteral Systems in the Dorsal and Sacral regions.

We know embryologically, the bones represent the last structural development and, as growth continues, the vital organs of the body are built on, or into, the solid frame-work that is taking shape and we see by this that the main functions of the body structural frame-work are those of support – protection – and mobility.

On the other hand, coincident with the body development, we have the gradual development of the shape and physiological function of the organs, which, at this stage, undoubtedly, largely determine the form of the growing skeletal structure.

Hence the accepted law – Function determines Structure in Development, and this state of affairs continues throughout the intra uterine life until after the child is born and locomotion begins.

Just as the Spine embryologically represents the centre from which all those vital forces necessary to motivity and animation or functional integrity arise, so it is also the centre of body mechanics and, when we follow its skeletal development, it becomes obvious to us why the dorsal and sacral regions are spoken of as the primary curves, their object being, as previously stated, through their frame-work to make room for support, protection, and to regulate the development of the thoracic and pelvic viscera.

These curves then, in view of the nature of their employment, must represent the alignment of certain groups of solidity, and we find that nature has provided for this solidity in the make-up and shape of the bodies of the vertebrae and developing ribs on the one hand, and the sacrum and innominate bones on the other, giving us the commencement of the definite curves of the spinal column and furnishing us with a foundation upon which we base our theory of the eventual posture of the body being laid in the child spine before it attempts to assume the erect position.

Carrying this a little further, we know that, from the time the child is born until it stands erect, is the most critical period of its life. The change from infancy to childhood is beset with innumerable difficulties which are mainly the result of a mother's lack of foresight, or knowledge. All, or most of these difficulties could be avoided if the mother took a little trouble to understand another of nature's axioms – namely:

'Mobility is the fundamental law of life'.

Normality of structure and function must be positive at this stage because the normal condition of the body depends on the integrity of its structure and the normality of movement in the structure.

We can best comprehend this by visualising the common procedure from the time the baby is born.

If a child is made to lie on its back until it can sit up, and is then kept sitting until it can stand, the whole structure of the body is likely to be altered and the child grow up with postural defects because, in the first place, the continual position on the back would result in circulatory congestion of the spinal cord and its meninges through pressure and gravitation, following which would come atonicity of the muscles, especially those of the Erector Spinae group, and a general muscular inequality which, when the child did sit up, would allow the body to droop forward and crowd in on the viscera, giving rise to impaired functional activities and malalignment in the structural adjustment.

Consequently, when the child stands, or attempts to do so, there is an unequal distribution of the body weight with a resultant inability to maintain the antero-posterior equilibrium and the child, in attempting to overcome this handicap, puts out such constant muscular effort, that any reserve energy it is likely to have is quickly taken up and there is very little left for development purposes, organic or otherwise.

Eventually, with the child standing on its own, we find compensation taking place by way of pronation of the feet, sagging knees, tilted pelvis, a posterior rounded spine, drooping shoulders and backward stress tension of the neck and head, the whole presenting a clinical picture of postural deformity with profound nervous exhaustion and consequent ill-health, thus laying the basis for modification and alteration in the behaviour of the physiological movements in the adult spine.

Obviously then, to prevent this we must lay down certain regulations to see that the physical laws of balance are encouraged as much as possible, and in this respect Nature again provides us with the necessary material to oppose the solidity of its primary posterior curves by giving us two areas of excessive flexibilty as accessory physical supports.

These areas we know as the lumbar and cervical regions, their curves are concave anterior in oppositon to the posterior convexity of the primary ones, their direction being almost entirely due to the size, shape and degree of consistency, in the development of the intervertebral discs and cartilages; their function as accessory physical supports must be developed and maintained by the child's own volitional movements and, in view of this, must represent flexibility in the ultimate determination of the definite curves of the erect posture.

Therefore, we have two groups of curves – the primary posterior curves which represent the definite curves of the spinal column and make their appearance during the embryonic stage, their shape being due to the bodies of the vertebrae and subsequent bony development and their function that of protection and regulation of the development of visceral life.

The secondary anterior curves which represent the definite curves of the erect posture and which make their appearance between infancy and childhood, their shape being due to the size and condition of the intervertebral discs and cartilages and their function that of accessory physical support.

The resultant of these two groups of curves should represent a balance between solidity and fluidity with the rigidity of the primary curves compensated for by the flexibility of the secondary ones.

The whole working in combination with each other represents the spinal accommodation to the erect posture of the body, and should provide us with perfect structural alignment and physiological adjustment, the co-ordination of which is a necessary qualification for a perfect functional activity.

To sum up:

Therefore, we find that the normal balance of the spine in the individual body depends on:

(i) the size and shape of the vertebral bodies;
(ii) the consistency and degree of elasticity in the intervertebral discs, and variations in both, through:
   (a) changes in tension of ligaments, cartilages and muscle, or
   (b) modification in the amount of blood or lymph in or to a particular area.

With this short summary of the development of the spine in mind, it is easy to see how any produced alteration either from postural abuse or direct or indirect trauma can effect changes in direction and behaviour of the physiological movements.

These physiological movements of the spine are subject to various laws, rules and regulations which must always be borne in mind when any attempt is made to apply them to the body in an effort to trace the pathway of lesion production and, in reversing that pathway in correction.

Perhaps a little recapitulation at this stage might help us to remember that:

Easy Normal Flexion or Neutral represents – a vertebra in its normal position within a curve with the weight resting on the body and intervertebral discs, and with the facets free to move in any direction.

Flexion represents – an increase of the normal curve in any given area of the spine.

Extension represents – a decrease of the normal curve in any given area of the spine.

Rotation represents – the direction of movement around a vertical axis to the right or left of the midline as indicated by the position of the body of the vertebrae.

Sidebending – represents the position assumed by the vertebra in side-bending to the right or left of the midline.

Rotation and Sidebending are complementary irrespective of which movement has precedence.

The two most important parts of the vertebrae which constitute the control of all spinal mobility are the bodies of the vertebrae and the articulating facets.

The body and intervertebral discs support and control the movements and distribution of the superimposed weights when the spinal curves are in the position of easy normal flexion or neutral.

The articulating facets, on the other hand, guide and control the direction of movement when any area or spinal curve is taken out of its normal and into extension or hyperflexion.

While we are on this subject of terminology, I think it would be well worth while to try to clarify what appears to be a new jargon coming into being, either that or else the old terminology seems to have been thrown hither and thither until it is hardly intelligible to anyone.

For some reason the Americans seem to dislike some of the old-fashioned words like sidebending or sidebending-rotation or rotation-sidebending, so they have substituted, contracted and added until they have evolved what (we are asked to believe) is the ideal terminolgy and which I must quote to you in case you take up the study of these physiological movements, and have need to refer to the latest American literature. About 15-20 years ago they slipped in the term Lateral Flexion as a substitute for sidebending, which I, personally, think is clumsy and unnecessary, but around six or seven years ago they decided on a complete change and (6) H.V. Hoover and C.R. Nelson in the name of the Academy of Applied Osteopathy in a combined lecture on the *'Effects of Gravitational Forces on Structure'* announced this change in the following manner:

"Parenthetically, at this point, it is necessary to insert definitions of terms which the Academy faculty has adopted from Dorland's dictionary for use in the discussion of the physiological movements of the spine with the hope of avoiding the confusion engendered by various definitions of the words flexion and extension in previous discussions.

> Antexion is forward bending of the spine and pelvis in relation to the lower extremities.
>
> Postexion is backward bending of the spine and pelvis in relation to the lower extremities.
>
> These replace respectively flexion and extension of the spine as defined by the anatomists and used in the Colleges in teaching the physiological movements.

Latexion is the motion of the spine combining lateral flexion to one side and rotation of the body of the vertebra to the other side. It occurs when the spine moves from easy normal in any direction, except into Antexion or Postexion.

Rotexion is the motion of the spine combining rotation of the body of the vertebra and lateral flexion to the same side. It occurs when the spine moves to one side or the other in an area of extension or marked flexion.

N.B. – When the terms flexion and extension are used in discussing spinal physiology, they are applied to given areas of the spine specifically named at the time as 'extension at the 5th thoracic' or 'flexion in the cervical area.'

Flexion of a given area of the spine is defined as an increase in the concavity of the normal antero-posterior curve of that area. Extension of a given area of the spine is defined as a decrease in that concavity of the normal antero-posterior curve of that area."

These last three sentences are exactly as Fryette stated in his original paper and as Littlejohn repeatedly taught, and negatives all the differences that have supposed to have existed since then. So why the change?

If you have unravelled this you will realise it is good old-fashioned English dressed up in ultra modern style.

We do not have to understand this to like it, but we must know it so that we can comprehend any of the literature written on this subject by any expert in the profession.

However, for myself, I prefer to reduce problems like this to the simplest possible form, and I hope I shall be able to demonstrate to you that understanding of these physiological movements need not be as complicated as they appear to be.

The spine, as we know, is a very mobile mechanism, and if anything goes wrong it shows itself by way of a defect in this mobility – therefore, we must have some formula to enable us to determine what is wrong and why, and how this defect in mobility occurred.

The answer is to be found in the four basic movements of the spine from the neutral position. But what, we may ask, is the neutral position? It can best be defined as the position in which any area or curve of the spine is found with the articulating facets oscillating between flexion and extension. In other words, these facets are 'idling' – waiting to go into action if and when that particular area of curve is taken out of this neutral position.

The four basic movements, therefore, from the neutral position are the simple movements of Flexion and Extension and the compound movements of Flexion-Sidebending-Rotation and Extension-Rotation-Sidebending. (6) Dr Littlejohn defined these movements in this manner:

Simple Flexion – when the physiological curve is increased that represents flexion of that curve.

Simple Extension – when the physiological curve is decreased that represents extension of that curve.

Flexion-Sidebending-Rotation in that sequence of motion occurs when the superimposed weight is resting mainly on the bodies of the vertebrae and the articulating facets are disengaged or idling – if any sidebending is attempted in this position the bodies try to crawl out from under this ill-balanced load and move into the produced convexity.

Extension-Rotation-Sidebending in that sequence of motion occurs when any area of the spine is moved into flexion or extension and the articulating facets take over the functions of guiding and controlling motion in that position. If sidebending is attempted under these conditions then the bodies of the vertebrae are moved or forcibly rotated into the concavity of the produced curve.

There is a fifth movement often mentioned which is designated a Hyper Flexion-Rotation-Sidebending lesion and which, in effect, behaves very similarly to the Extension-Rotation-Sidebending lesion, but it is difficult for the spinal mechanism to support this form of distortion and, while it is theoretically possible to produce this type of lesion, for all practical purposes it can be disregarded in treatment. In fact, Dr Fryette (7) says he has never seen a lesion of this extreme flexion type with the bodies rotated to the concavity in 50 years of practice. Therefore, to all intents and purposes we have only two laws (apart from straight extension and flexion) operating and covering the physiological movements of the spine.

Let us examine the first law – that covering the large curvatures from functional to organic scoliosis – the group lesion – the lesion that arises from the introduction into the articulation of a force (mainly gravitational or a direct blow) which is permissible but, cumulatively results in an excess of that permitted motion and goes beyond the ability of the soft tissues to resist it. This is the Flexion-Sidebending-Rotation lesion involving mainly the bodies of the vertebra and intervertebral discs. It is a passively produced condition following in the main on postural abuse in a facet free area.

With the articulating facets free to move, and on side-bending being introduced, the bodies of the vertebrae move over to the convex side of the curve produced, which curve increases simultaneously upwards and downwards from the central point (of the original side-bending) followed by an equal increase in gross rotation towards the convexity and with total movement towards the lateral side of the central or median line. In other words this is the method of development in scoliosis.

As this side-bending and rotation increases, the inferior facet on the concave side is forced to approximate closer to the superior facet below and the inferior facet on the convex side is compelled to separate to the limit of capsular strain from the superior facet below.

This means that any treatment given which aims at reduction of these produced curves must first give attention to the restoration of flexion and extension before attempting to reduce the gross Side-bending and Rotation.

The second law covers that of the single or small group lesion. The 'Still Lesion' – the Lesion on which osteopathy has built its reputation over the past 70 years, and which is so named in honour of our founder – Dr Andrew Taylor Still. This Lesion results from the introduction of a force into the joint in complete violation of the permitted mechanics.

This is the Extension-Rotation-Sidebending lesion and it involves mainly the articulating facets, ligaments and cartilages. It is an actively produced condition following in the main on any form of voluntary exercise superimposed upon a facet locked area. Given the above conditions, the spinal column takes on the characteristics of a flexible rod and must by torsion rotate before it can sidebend. Therefore, this law states, that when any area or curve of the spine is moved into extension when the facets are locked by forced tissue rigidity or – theoretically into hyperflexion, when the facets are locked by bony contact, of Spinous Processes or Facets, and side-bending is introduced, the bodies of the vertebrae rotate towards the concavity of the curve produced with rotation preceding side-bending.

When rotation and side-bending both move towards the concavity of the produced curve, the vertebra as a whole remains within the orbit of the median or central line.

As this lesion involves mainly the articulating facets, ligaments and cartilages, any treatment which aims at correction of the maladjustments must be of an articulatory nature and must, therefore, be introduced by way of rotation.

These physiological movements as outlined are based upon the ideal in spinal mechanics but, as we all know, our patients provide us with experience which is gained at the expense of the exception rather than the rule, but nevertheless these laws do operate as stated, although they may make us work harder.

It is seldom we see a normal spine; at the same time, apart from gross scoliosis, we seldom also see a spinal curve that has completely reversed itself. The reversed lumbar curve, which is so common, with its loss of the normal lordosis, reacts to the physiological movements just the same except that the distance travelled before trouble overtakes is considerably shorter – remember the case who just leaned forward to pick up the soap –

he was standing in front of the wash basin and swears he did not bend his back but just leaned forward – his reactive pain is mostly sharp and he feels stuck – can't, or is afraid to move – there is no pelvic sideshift but a mild pelvic torsional rotation.

Here is your Extension-Rotation-Sidebending lesion to the side of reaching forward – the spinous process moved well over to the opposite side, painful to palpation on its convex side, pain is experienced on deep pressure over the post inferior transverse process which has moved downward, backward and medialward on the concave side with all the tissues crowded together.

There are many more definite diagnostic points, but I feel I cannot take up too much time on these, but for those interested I would strongly recommend for study the article by (8) H.V. Hoover and C.R. Nelson on the *'Basic Physiological Movements of the Spine'*, published in the Academy Year Book for 1950, pages 63-66. This gives a full and comprehensive outline of this subject.

Now just a word as to the Correction of Lesions.

The structural maladjustments that we recognise as abnormal are produced or maintained by changes in the soft or supporting tissues. The removal of this pathology can be carried out by following a number of procedures such as – Muscle and Ligamentous stretch, Articulation and Specific Bony correction.

Without undermining the importance of the first two, I think we would quicken our results if more detailed attention was paid to the third procedure, bearing in mind that the first two are essentially preparatory methods.

The need for this specific application of corrective force is recognised when we consider that a force misapplied to a region of the spine sufficient to move the lesioned segments will produce injury to the normal tissues, while a force sufficient to move the normal articulations and yet not produce injury will have little effect, if any, on the lesioned segments. Therefore, from the diagnosis of the abnormality we must determine exactly what motion or motions of the articulation need to be moved in correction.

If rotation is restricted, the major corrective force should be applied to normalise this motion. If extension of an area is the chief maladjustment, then increase in flexion is the first movement in correction specifically indicated.

A knowledge of the physiological movements of an area enables one to apply force in such a manner as to exact the maximum results with the minimum of effort on the part of the operator and patient.

Our object in specific technique is to reverse the pathology present in the quickest possible manner, and the most direct way to accomplish this is to trace the pathway of lesion production through the physiological movements and apply a force directly opposite to the motion or motions involved, with the end result that of normalisation.

(1) FRYETTE, H.H.
   Technique and Nomenclature, A.O.A. July, 1936

(2) LOVETT, R.W.
   Lateral Curvature of the Spine and Round Shoulders, 1907

(3) FRYETTE, H.H.
   Original manuscript of new book on Applied Technique, published 1954

(4) LITTLEJOHN, J. MARTIN
   Lectures, British School of Osteopathy, 1926, 27 and 28

(5) HALL, T. EDWARD
   Lectures, given at the British School of Osteopathy from 1931.

(6) HOOVER, H.V. and NELSON, C.R.
   Effects of Gravitational Forces on Structure, Academy of Applied Osteopathy, 1950

(7) FRYETTE, H.H.
   Year Book, Academy of Applied Osteopathy, 1950

(8) HOOVER, H.V. and NELSON, C.R.
   Basic Physiological Movements of the Spine, Academy Year Book, 1950

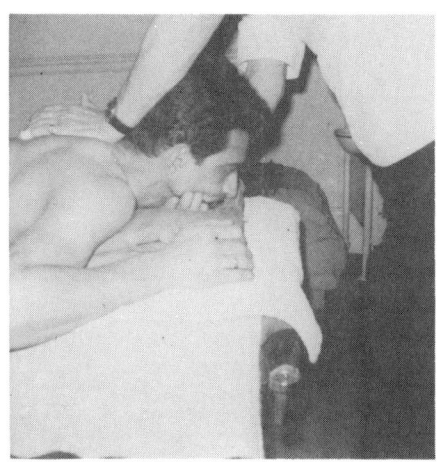

UPPER RIBS
Shoulder blades spread
Chin stablilised.
Direct thrust on angle of rib.

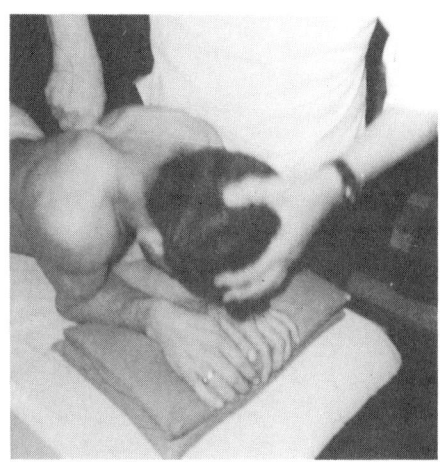

DORSALS
Head stablilised.
Shoulder blades spread.
Direct thrust on vertebrae.

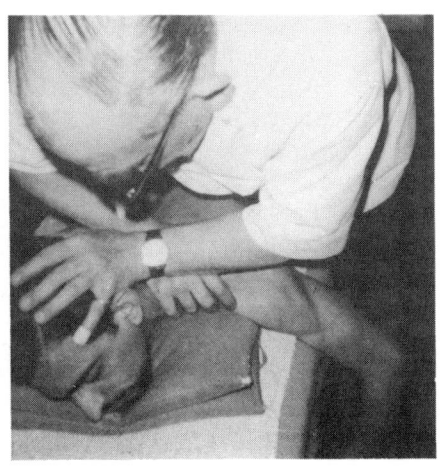

FIRST RIB
Cross hands.
Neck and rib thrust.

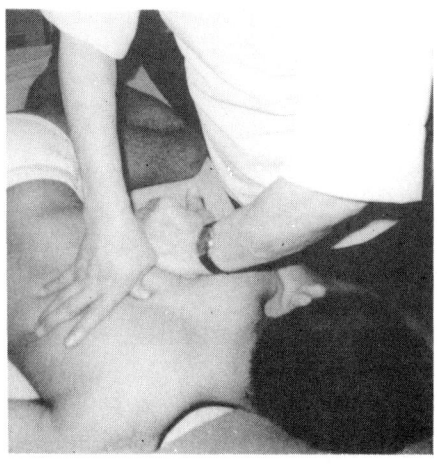

UPPER DORSALS AND RIBS
Cross hands thrust.

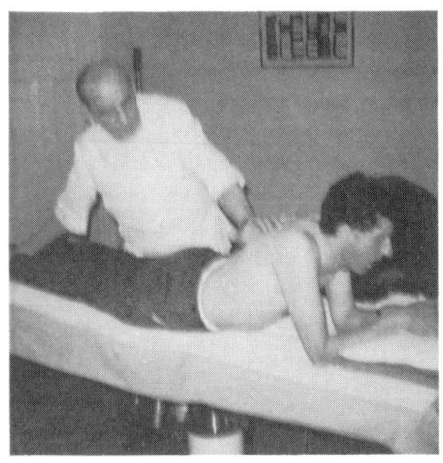

UPPER RIBS
Long arm thrust.

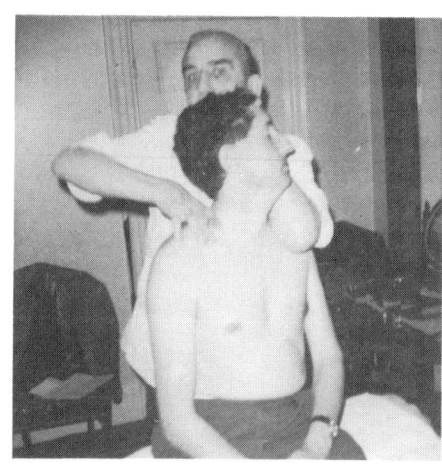

FIRST RIB
Patient sitting. Method 1

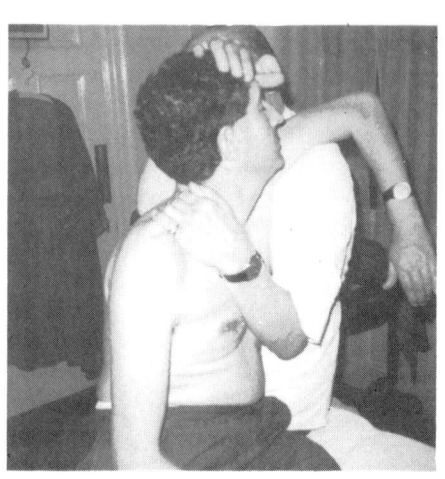

FIRST RIB
Patient sitting. Method 2

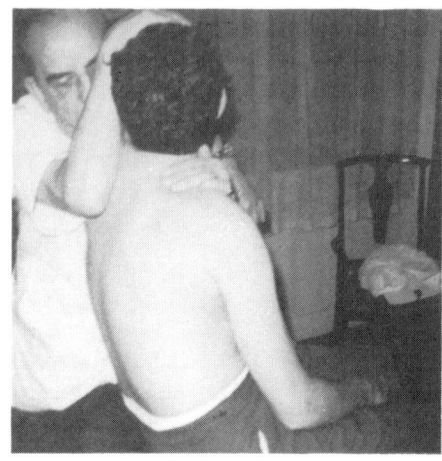

FIRST RIB
*Patient sitting. Method 2
(Reverse angle)*

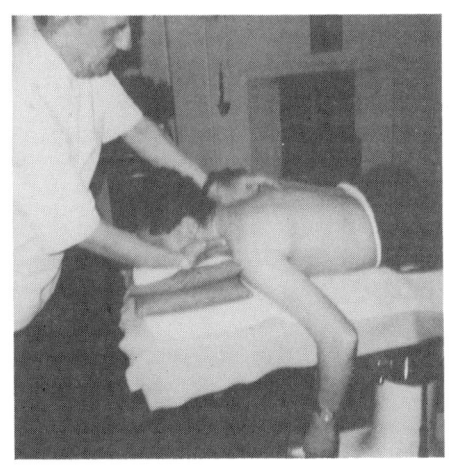

FIRST RIB
Chin pivot technique.
Position

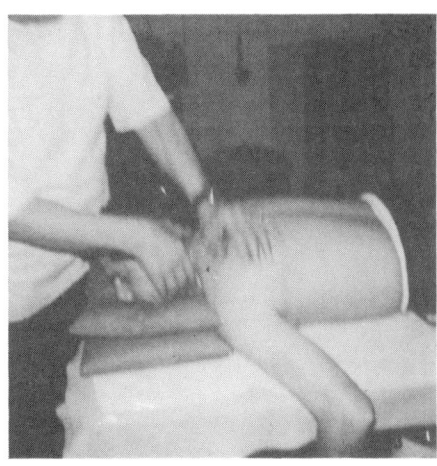

FIRST RIB
Chin pivot technique.
Thrust

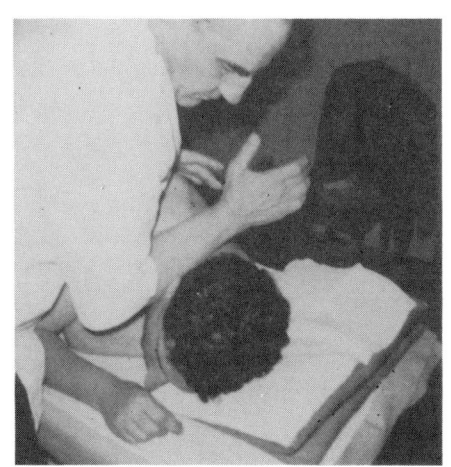

FIRST RIB
Patient on side.

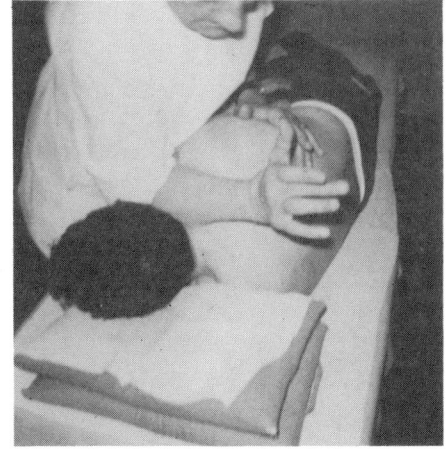

FIRST RIB
Patient on side.
(Reverse angle)

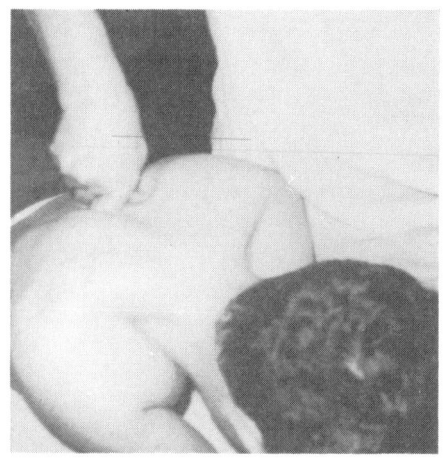

UPPER RIBS
Stabilising spinous process.

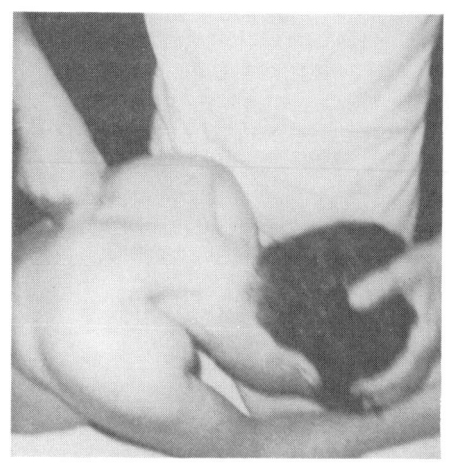

UPPER RIBS
Moving the upper column.

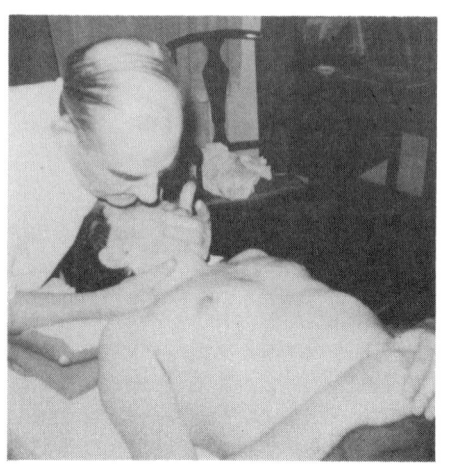

FIRST RIB
Patient supine.

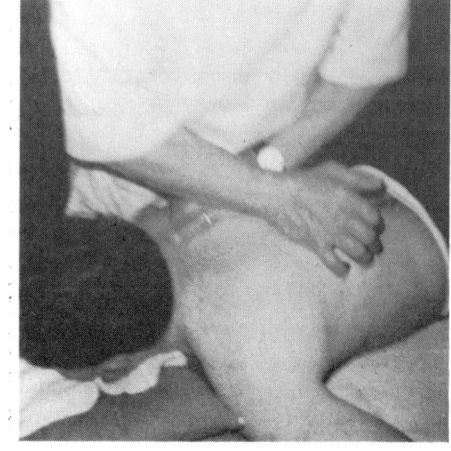

RIBS
Cross hands thrust.

MECHANICS OF LESION DIAGNOSIS IN THE PELVIS

When I was asked to give this demonstration of pelvic technique I consented to do so provided that I was given an opportunity to explain briefly the interpretation of pelvic mechanics which I favour in my own practice. Before doing this, I would like to quote a passage from Dr Castlio's book on the Principles of Osteopathy which, to my mind, is absolutely fundamental to anyone interested in teaching osteopathic technique.

"Osteopathic technique cannot be acquired by a study of books; it must be learned by personal demonstration and application. If a student is shown a series of manipulations designed to correct a lesion without having the principles upon which they are based made clear to him, he can do nothing else but blindly copy the movements. He will be unable to improvise those slight variations in technique that different patients and varied circumstances demand. He will do awkward and inefficient work."

Unfortunately, it appears that students are apt not to be interested in the principles of technique; the eternal cry is "show me how", and but little interest is shown in the reason "why". We cannot hope to practise osteopathic technique without knowing the principles upon which the technique is based, and it is only when these principles are thoroughly grasped that "specific" technique can occupy its rightful place in our daily practice.

Another fundamental point which is often overlooked in our teaching is that 75% of technique is diagnosis. If this simple truth was more generally understood, much laborious and ineffective treatment would be avoided, for it is safe to say that osteopathic treatment which is not preceded by careful diagnosis can be successful only by chance. Moreover, much of the controversy on the principles of pelvic mechanics and of the techniques based thereon could be eliminated if more attention were given to these two fundamental points.

It is my opinion, therefore, that diagnosis of low back conditions, and especially of the pelvis, should only be made after a general routine examination which, by elimination of all extraneous factors, will enable you to pinpoint the primary lesions and to select the appropriate techniques for adjustment. We must remember that a large proportion of apparent pelvic lesions are secondary or compensatory to conditions of strain or sprain arising from causes outside the pelvic ring, that is, structural or functional pathology above or below. For example, below the pelvic ring we have such things as foot and knee conditions, primary short leg, acetabular limitation of internal or external rotation (the former often accompanying primary short leg or posterior ilium) fractures and altered angles of the neck of the femur, Varus and Valgus conditions, psoas affections, etc. Above, there may be curvatures giving rise to torsion in the erector spinae muscles and the spinal column which, however, is counteracted by the persistence of the shoulders in facing frontwards and the ability of the pelvis to counter-rotate on the heads of the femora within the acetabula. Again, there may be psoas or ilio-psoas lesions with intense unilateral muscle spasm, as in acute sciatica and lumbago, giving rise to that typical side shift of the pelvis with which we are all familiar. Pathology in the lumbo-sacral area such as bone anomalies, sacralization or lumbarization which may be unilateral or bilateral, dorsal facets which are usually unilateral, may also be producing effects. Lesions, even as high as the head, may in certain circumstances be important, as, for instance, defective eyesight affecting one eye more than the other, as in cases of advanced diplopia. It is illuminating to reflect that Schwab lists at least 12 basic causes for the primary short leg alone. Errors of locomotion, of which a long list could be made, are frequently the primary cause of pelvic lesions. Perhaps the commonest of these arises from a high arch on one side and a flat foot on the other. Another external cause is psoas fibrositis. These patients are usually in great pain, having lesions mostly of the second and third lumbar, and are bent forwards or forwards and laterally according to the type of lesion present, which is commonly unilateral but can be bilateral. Any of these conditions can produce or give rise to strain, sprain or torsion of the sacro-iliac ligaments and so cause pain, especially when the strain is sufficient to induce periostitis at the site of ligamentous attachment.

If these extraneous conditions are left unaltered for long enough they naturally lead to definite maladjustment of the pelvic articulations but they are, in the main, outside the pelvic ring proper, as their history and the examination of the patient will confirm, and they should be dealt with by attention to the initial cause, following which most of the apparent bony lesions will be found to have been eliminated. A common example of this is the easily corrected innominate lesion which just as easily recurs unless we look elsewhere for the primary cause. All these extraneous conditions may be conveniently grouped under the heading of *'Disturbance of Mobile Physiology'* following on some form of predisposing functional misuse. This in turn may be due to indirect strain or sprain of the ligaments within the pelvic ring, including those of the lumbo-sacral articulation, to referred and/or reflex signs affecting the pelvis from irritation of the lumbar plexus and its branches anywhere within the lumbar area, and sometimes to disease or infection such as tuberculosis, arthritis, ankylosing spondylitis, etc., giving rise to inflammatory conditions.

Leaving aside these conditions with causes external to the pelvis, we come to those in which there is actual disturbance or maladjustment of the articular structure of the pelvic ring, that is to say, actual alteration in the alignment of the auricular surfaces to each other, and it is with these that we are mainly concerned. The mechanics of the pelvis and of the lumbo-sacral articulations have long been the subject of much debate and we are still very far from reaching any final decision as to what goes on in the pelvis. Much of the uncertainty which exists concerning sacro-iliac lesions is due to the lack of facilities for research on the pelvis, both as to its constituent parts and as to the movements of the pelvic girdle in locomotion. Until our knowledge of the physics involved in the physiology of the sacro-iliac and sacro-lumbar articulations is increased, and the many theories in existence are subjected to clinical tests, there must be a certain amount of empiricism in our methods.

There have been many interpretaions of the mechanics of the pelvis over the years, notably those of Fryette and Pratt in 1914, that of Schwab in 1932-3, and that of Clark as far back as 1906. Many other authorities have made contributions to the apparent solution of the pelvic problem, and most are agreed that when the true Still lesion is found in the pelvis, that is to say, a maladjusted articulation of the sacro-iliac joint and not merely referred ligamentous strain, even the one-man technique has proved much more specific and effective when based on the theory of movement around the vertical and horizontal arms of the auricular surfaces of the articulation.

According to Schwab, "These investigations appear to suggest that movement in the sacro-iliac articulation occurs in definite directions. These movements are limited in extent, yet there must be present a degree of freedom sufficient to allow for easy and rapid movement, and were it not for these vertical and horizontal auricular surfaces acting as orderly directing agencies, then sacral pathology, and the mechanics of the sacrum, would appear to be complete chaos." To clarify the position, therefore, we must consider the movements of the sacrum and the ilium as separate entities, the primary movement being that of the sacrum on the ilium, and the innominates moving secondarily on the sacrum. The auricular surfaces are roughly 'L' shaped. In the standing or sitting position the 'L' would appear as lying on its back, that is to say, the upright of the 'L' becomes the horizontal arm reaching out from the posterior-inferior spine nearly at right angles with the erect position of the body, while the base of the 'L' becomes the vertical upper arm and is, to all intents and purposes, parallel with the erect position of the body. Both these arms join anteriorly to form an angle at the apex. The posterior-superior spine of the ilium is found behind, usually slightly below, this apex. It is this shape and position of the two arms, together with the apex, which form the complete auricular surface of the sacrum or ilia, and the position in relation to these of the posterior-superior spine which, when correctly visualised, add so much to the correct diagnosis and treatment of sacro-iliac lesions. It is this visualisation in the varied positions of standing, sitting, prone and supine which is a difficult art to acquire but which, when acquired, makes sacro-iliac diagnosis and treatment more interesting and successful.

Schwab states that "As a general rule, the external forces sufficient to cause primary pathology within the sacro-iliac mechanism are usually extreme in degree." This view is supported by Clark who says, "Considerable force is usually exerted in the production of all lesions of this joint. This is because of the size, shape and character of the articulations. The joint itself is injured to a greater extent than the joints involved in vertebral lesions, for the reason that the sacro-iliac joint is designed for movement which is limited but must be maintained. The original force does not necessarily require to be of great extent but it does require to be of high velocity to enable it to forestall the natural protection offered by the neuro-muscular mechanism." A typical example of high velocity force is furnished by turning and spraining of the ankle, which penetrates the muscle guard in the foot by the speed of the turnover, which implies more damage to ligaments than to muscles. The same thing applies to sacro-iliac lesions. We must remember, therefore, that the articulations of the pelvis are not maintained by muscles, but solely by their intrinsic ligaments. These are: the anterior sacro-iliac ligaments, the anterior common ligament, the posterior sacro-iliac ligaments, the interosseous ligaments, the transverse and oblique ligaments and the accessory and stabilising ligaments, such as the ilio-lumbar, sacro-tuberous and sacro-spinous ligaments. This means that there is no appreciable muscle support, but strong intrinsic and accessory ligamentous support, giving us a weight-bearing articulation which is only slightly moveable. The trunk weight is supported through the sacro-iliac joints almost entirely by ligaments. Injury, therefore, most frequently affects these ligamentous structures, especially at their osseous attachments.

In any given case, certain of these ligaments are affected more than others, according to which part of the articulation receives the impact of injury. This is because the forces producing the lesion are directed along one of the arms of the auricular surfaces round an axis the centre of which lies in the other arm. For example, in flexion of the sacrum the movement is directed anteriorly in the vertical arm round an axis in the horizontal arm. In the posterior conditions of the ilium the axis of movement is still in the lower arm, but the innominate travels backwards and superior. The anterior innominate, which has now become known as the up-posterior, takes place from an axis in the vertical arm and the movement occurs upwards and backwards along the horizontal arm. This gives the reason for the change in terminology because the innominate moves upward and backward. The reverse occurs in extension lesions of the sacrum (posterior sacrum). In these cases the axis of rotation arises in the short vertical arm, and the movement takes place in a forward direction along the horizontal arm. These principles are of great value in osteopathic diagnosis. Where the base of the sacrum is the moving element, and the movement is directed anteriorly by the surface of the vertical arm around an axis centred in the horizontal arm, then the maximum stress or strain will fall on the interosseous, the transverse and the short posterior sacro-iliac ligaments.

In chronic lesions of this area, symptoms of pain and tenderness are usually referred to the area of the gluteus medius muscle. It is remarkable that nearly all objective and subjective signs are confined within the area above the posterior-superior spine, and the strain falls on the ligaments and the gluteus medius whether the sacrum has moved forward between the ilia or the ilium has moved back on the vertical arm. It is commonly found on examination that when there is a pain point at the superior sacro-iliac articulation, the lesion proves to be an anterior sacrum, or posterior innominate, whereas when the sacrum is extended or the innominate is up-posterior, we have the typical lesion which is mostly present in specific and painful sciatica, irrespective, it would seem, of the position assumed by the lumbar vertebrae. It would be of value to establish statistically the proportion of sciatica cases in which the pain is on the "long side" indicating an up-posterior innominate. In the chronic lesion involving this extended sacrum and/or up-posterior innominate, similar signs and symptoms are found that in most cases give rise to tenderness and pain which are referred to the gluteus maximus and the area below the posterior-superior spine. All of these points are of the utmost importance in differential diagnosis.

Up to this point we have reviewed the basic movements of flexion and extension of the sacrum and of the innominates, but we must not lose sight of the secondary movements, which are of special importance in the case of sacro-iliac lesions. The primary movements of flexion and extension, and the secondary movements of side-bending and rotation apply as much to the pelvis as they do, for instance, to the elbow joint. The sacrum is the most common cause of sacro-iliac pathology, but simple bilateral flexion of the sacrum is a rare condition, and there is more usually a combination of flexion and rotation round a vertical axis in the sacrum. In practice we have to try to discover which is the primary and which is the secondary of these movements.

In kypho-lordotic spines, and in straight spines, whether in flexion or extension, the iliac crests are found to be relatively level, but the sacrum appears to have moved backwards or forwards. On the other hand, in primary innominate conditions, that is, ilio-sacral lesions, the sacrum is usually level but the iliac crests are uneven. The straightforward movements of the sacrum on the ilia and of the ilia on the sacrum take place as a result of the mechanics I have endeavoured to outline. The effect on the tissues in the area surrounding the sacro-iliac articulation is much the same in both types of lesion, except that when the innominate is in lesion as a result of a secondary or compensatory condition, there is usually a rotation or twist of the sacrum with the innominate moving forward on the one side and backward on the other. In these circumstances there is a torsional stress and tension on certain groups of muscles in the lower extremity arising from the enforced alteration of the resting plane of the femur in the acetabulum. This means that the pelvic compensation affects the internal and external rotators and is a powerful factor in the apparent lengthening and shortening of the legs. As a preliminary in the diagnosis of this more complicated type of pelvis, it is, therefore, necessary to relax these muscles thoroughly. Many complications of the various movements are possible in the chronic case, but many of the difficulties of diagnosis can be overcome by a process of elimination, and if we bear in mind these pelvic mechanics, it should be possible to arrive at a relatively true picture of the essential lesion.

ROUTINE EXAMINATION

Having described the intra-articular maladjustments, we are now ready to describe the routine examination of the patient, in which my procedure is as follows:

The patient should be undressed except for a pair of shorts and is asked to stand with both heels together and hands and arms hanging loosely by his side. Visual note should then be taken of the gross contours of the body as a whole and the spine in particular. Note the symmetry or asymmetry in the levels of the shoulders and iliac crests. In a typical case of primary short leg, if the patient is not too fat the iliac crest on the side of the shortening will generally appear to be slightly lower. The lumbar area will give the impression of being convex to the same side and the shoulder on that side higher.

The overall picture is the same in the case of a primary posterior sacro-iliac lesion except that the shoulder appears lower. When these gross conditions have been noted, the operator should place his hands over the posterior part of the pelvis with the thumbs touching the iliac crests just above the posterior-superior spines and the little fingers resting on top and lateralwards of the great trochanters. Visual comparison will show the hand on the side of the short leg to be lower both at the crest and at the trochanters, except in cases of fractures or similar conditions of the neck or head of the femur, when it is common to find the trochanters symmetrical in height from the ground level but the crest on the short side lower. This condition must, of course, be confirmed by enquiry into the history and further examination.

The next step in the primary short leg examination is to ask the patient to flex the trunk forward upon the hips keeping the knees braced and the arms hanging loosely from the shoulders. It is a mistake to allow the patient to rest his hands on the thighs. When the maximum normal degree of trunk flexion has been reached, the palms of the operator's hands should be placed over the pelvis with the thumbs touching each other over the lower lumbar spinous processes. The hands should then be allowed to slide laterally, keeping contact with the skin until they slide over the great trochanters. This movement can be repeated a few times and an impression can thus be obtained of the general tilt of the pelvis towards the short side and of the gluteal muscles which appear less well rounded under palpation than those on the opposite side. The findings can often be corroborated, if there is any doubt, by going to the patient's head and looking down his flexed trunk to the pelvis.

The examination has so far taken place with the patient standing and his heels together. If further confirmation of a primary short lower extremity is required, the patient can then be placed supine on the table and a check made of the difference in leg lengths aided, if necessary, by measurement with a tape. This is best done by taking a central fixed point at the xyphoid process and measuring down to and just beneath each anterior-superior spine. If there is a difference in length and the shorter line is on the same side as the shortened lower extremity, then, other things being equal, it is safe to assume that we have to deal with a functional short leg (up-anterior ilium). On the other hand, if the longer line is on the side of the short leg, we can assume that it a case of primary short leg. These measurement tests can be carried on down to the internal malleoli for reverse comparison with the above, and it may be as well here, while the patient is in the supine position, to apply the shortening and lengthening leg tests advocated by C.H. Downing.

The next step is to search the lower extremities for anything which could be classified as, or give rise to, a primary error of locomotion. Examine each articulation from foot to hip, comparing the two sides; note whether any fault found is functional or structural in origin and relate it to the pelvic structure above. In all cases of pain in the lower extremities, back and pelvis, you should of course apply all reflex tests, such as tests for plantar and ankle reactions, ankle clonus, knee and abdominal reflexes.

Next, with the patient in the prone position, note should be taken of any increase or decrease in gross body contours, particularly in relation to spinal curvatures and muscular and ligamentous tension. The test for psoas fibrositis is naturally made with the patient in this position. The operator should stand on the side opposite that to be tested. For example, standing on the right side of the patient, he should lean over and place his right hand firmly over the left sacro-iliac and take hold of the left thigh just above the knee with his left hand. The knee should not be flexed as this brings tension to bear on the quadriceps group of muscles and can result in a wrong psoas reading. He should then elevate the left extremity up to the point of resistance in extension while keeping the pelvis in contact with the table. In this test the extremity must be kept in the mid-line and not abducted or adducted. The greater the degree of psoas fibrositis the less extension and the greater resistance there will be. The test should be repeated on the opposite side and a comparison made. This should be followed by deep mobilising pressure over the lumbar spine to test the amount of extension and recoil in the area. It should be mentioned that all cases of true spondylosis will affect the functioning of the psoas to a greater or less degree. While the patient is still in this position, it is well to palpate for ligamentous and muscular tension in the lumbar and sacro-iliac areas, noting the findings for future reference and for correlation of other diagnostic points. Follow this by mobilisation tests of the pelvic articulations for comparison with the results of the palpation.

Finally, with the patient sitting on a surface which must be absolutely level, note the changes in spinal contours and muscular tension by comparison with the standing position. With the patient sitting erect, determine by palpation the relative positions of the anterior-superior spines, the iliac crests and the posterior-superior spines. If you have been able to eliminate all other conclusions by your examination up to this point, you can safely assume that certain lesions exist on the basis of your findings in respect of these three points. For example, if all three points (A.S.S., P.S.S. and iliac crest) appear to be elevated on one side in relation to the other and the sacrum gives the impression of being posterior on the *same* side, you can assume that there is a primary sacral lesion of side-bending and rotation forward on the *opposite* side. On the other hand, if only two of the three points appear to follow each other, you may assume that you are dealing with an ordinary innominate lesion of one kind or another.

Once this "routine elimination examination" has become an acquired habit, it is possible to run through it in from three to five minutes and it will add more than you realise to your experience and diagnostic ability in low back conditions, enabling you to work out your line of treatment and give a prognosis with equal confidence. It has been stated that such an examination is ponderous and impractical in private practice. If each lesion or finding is charted, this might be true, but if the examiner merely makes a mental note of the findings, he will find that once he becomes used to the routine, the examination will become more or less automatic, the negative findings being quickly discarded, and attention directed only to the few areas which are in trouble.

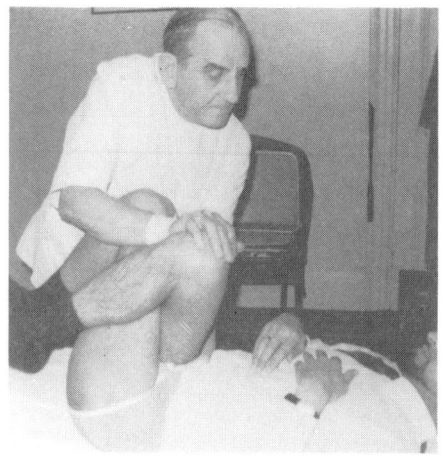

"NUT CRACKER" TECHNIQUE
Articulate lower lumbar and S.I. joint.

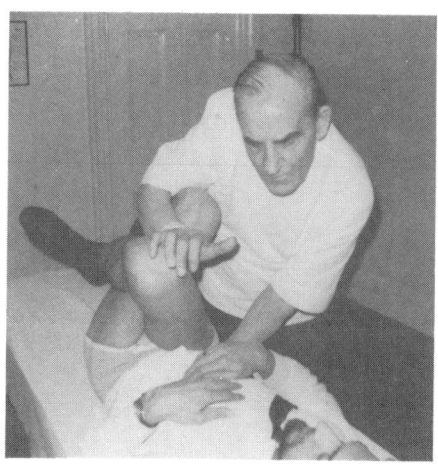

"NUT CRACKER" TECHNIQUE
Lower lumbar and S.I. joint. (Reverse view)

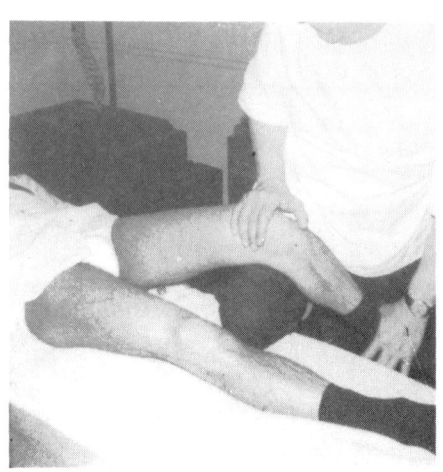

O.A. HIP
Internal and external rotation under traction.

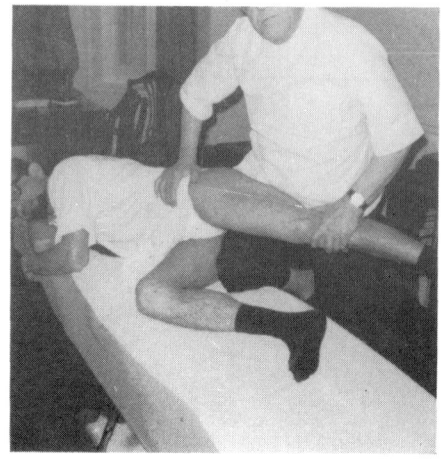

O.A. HIP
Gapping hip joint.

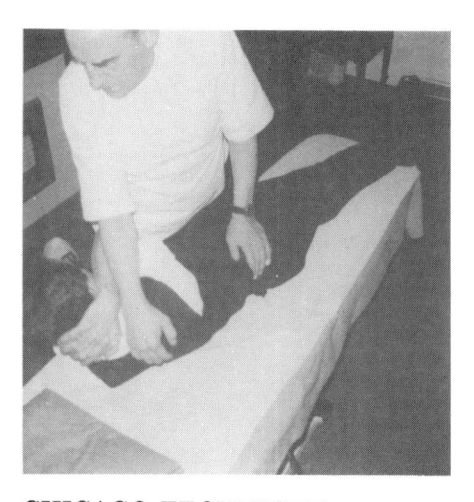

CHICAGO TECHNIQUE
Operator's position.
Iliac-crest stabilised with one arm.

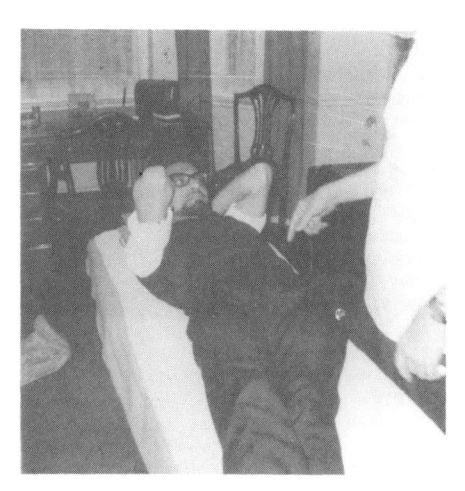

LUMBARS AND SACROILIAC
Chicago technique.
Patient's position.

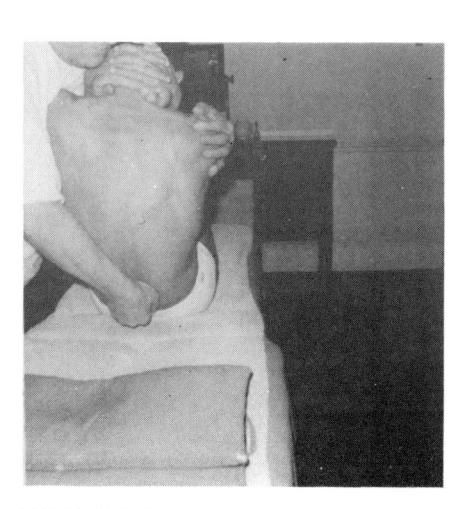

LUMBARS
Long roll technique.

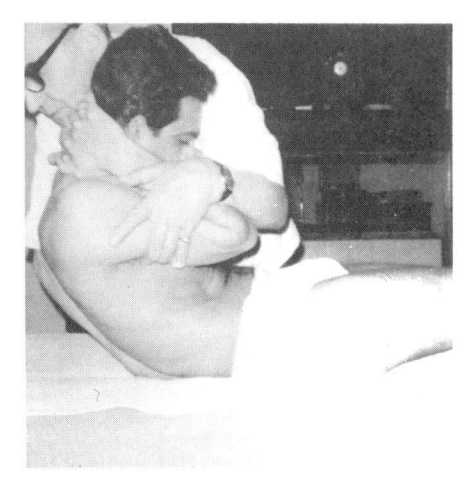

LUMBARS
Long roll technique.

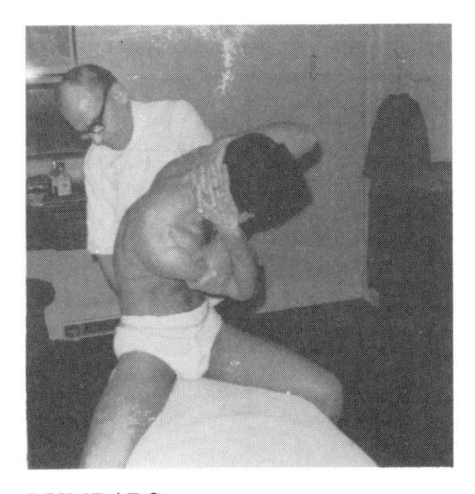

LUMBARS
Straddle technique.

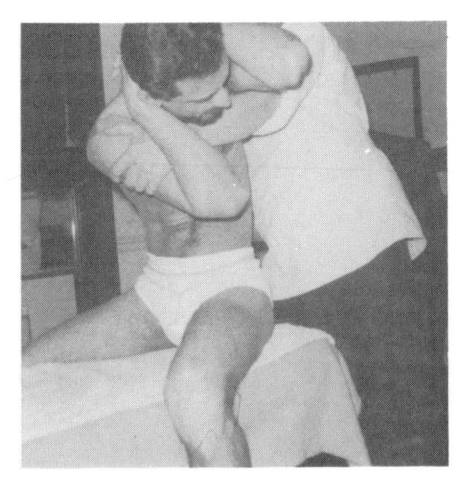

LUMBARS
Straddle technique.
(Reverse view)

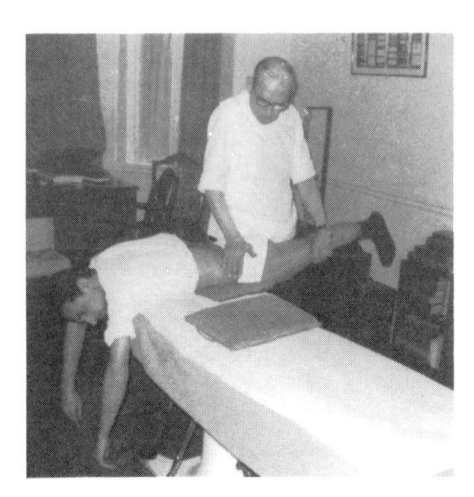

POSTERIOR ILIUM
Leg lever technique.

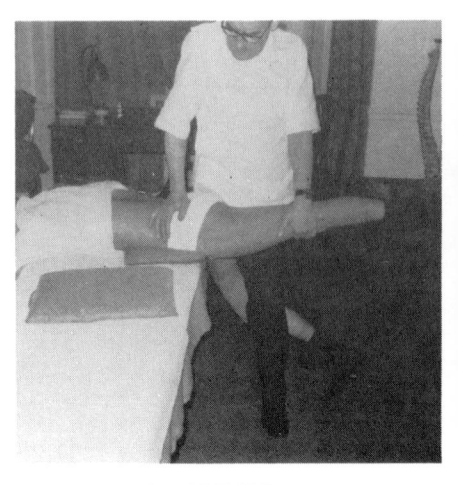

POSTERIOR ILIUM
Showing leg positioning.

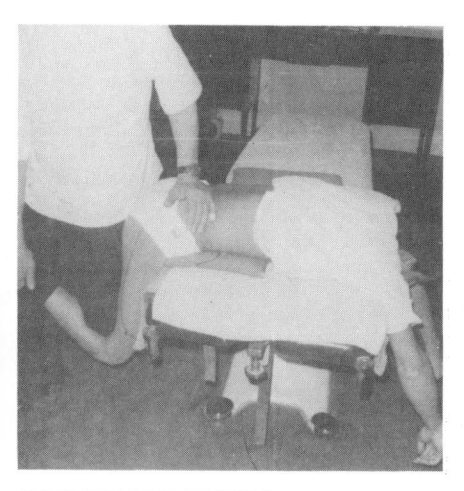

POSTERIOR ILIUM
Traction on bent leg technique.

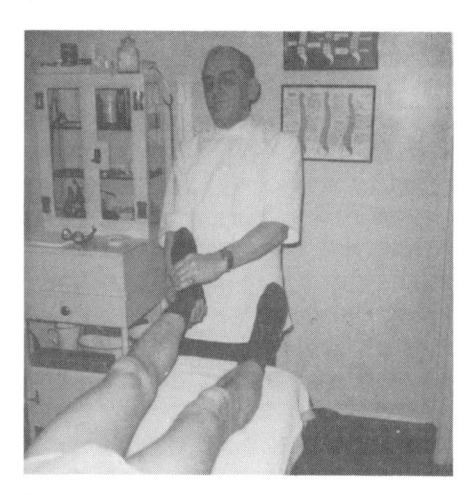

"LEG TUG" for posterior ilium.

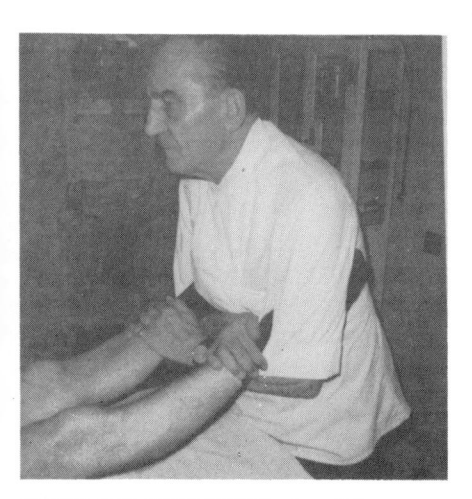

DOUBLE LEG PULL for S.I. joints.

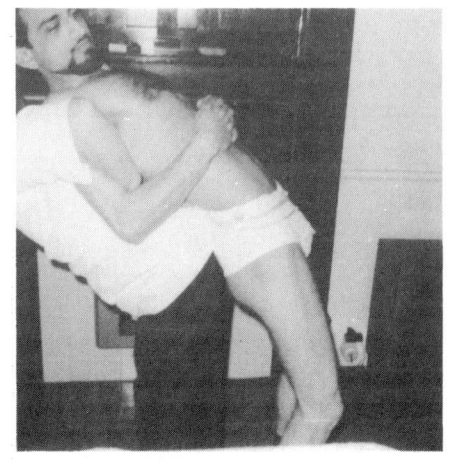

LOWER LUMBARS
Spondylolysthesis
"The Drop" technique.

DIAGNOSIS AND TREATMENT OF PSOAS MUSCLE CONDITIONS

To anyone interested in spinal mechanics and postural integrity, the subject matter of this talk should be of considerable interest.

Since student days, all of us have been interested, if only in a vague way, in the lumbar region. We have noted its flexibility, its stubbornness in correction, and its adaptive mechanism to gross structural changes existing anywhere in the body.

Low back pain, which represents a large percentage of all cases consulting an osteopath, has forced interest to be focussed upon this area. Most people present here today could no doubt suggest numerous different causes of low backache and pain and many have experienced how a general mobilisation, plus correction of lesions present, has effectually cleared the pathological signs; but how many have been interested in the accurate reasons producing this success and, again, how many have realised that a correction of 2-3-5 lumbar releases the psoas muscles and allows the maximum of relief to be obtained with a greater chance of recovery being permanent?

W.A. Schwab, D.O. says "In front of the lumbar area – antero-lateral – is located the only large prevertebral muscle mass. The complete understanding of the physiology of this muscle is the property of but a few. Psoas muscle pathology perverts lumbar physiology with ease, and is a common primary cause of malfunction in this region. Minor inflammations, fibrositis, and contractures of psoas muscle are impressively frequent and not always recognised as primary. This muscle also participates in the general pathologic pictures of primary lumbar maladjustment, and is then a secondary tissue condition."

Sir Colin McKenzie states "There is no muscle in the body whose action is of more diagnostic significance than that of the psoas magnus of man. Flexion of the thigh, due to reflex contraction of the ilio-psoas with relaxation and elongation of the gluteus maximus, is associated with many pathological conditions, such as the passage of a stone in the ureter, appendicitis and inflamed lymphatic glands in children, etc. The great value, however, of psoas contraction as a diagnostic help is in connection with disease of the lumbar vertebrae and joints, sacro-iliac joint, and the hip joint, with all of which it is in relation."

ANATOMY

Here it might be as well if we briefly reviewed the anatomical structure, relations and actions of this muscle.

According to McGregor, it is a long fusiform muscle, wider above and gradually narrowing towards its insertion in the hip joint. Its

attachments, 15 in number arise from:
- A. The antero-lateral portion of the bodies and the intra-vertebral discs of D.12 and all L. (Excepting possibly L.5.) (Author's note).
- B. The anterior surfaces and lower borders of the transverse processes of the lumbar vertebrae.
- C. The fibrous arches at the sides of the bodies of the lumbar vertebrae.

From the vertebral attachments, psoas crosses the pelvis and hip joint, diminishing in size to end in a tendon, combining its own fibres with those of the iliacus, and inserted into the lesser trochanter of the femur. This pull gives the flexion of the hip, and with the femur fixed, after the action of lumbar flexion, tilts the pelvis forwards.

According to Morris's treatise on anatomy, its relations are of the utmost importance. He says "The psoas major muscle lies lateral to the lumbar vertebrae and in front of the quadratus lumborum and intertransverse muscles. The psoas minor passes distally across its ventral surface. Both psoas muscles are crossed by the crura of the diaphragm. The kidney with its adipose capsule lies lateral to them opposite the first two lumbar vertebrae. For the rest, their fascia is covered ventro-laterally by retro-intestinal and retro-peritoneal tissue in which the vena cava inferior runs in front of them on the right side, the inferior mesenteric vein in front of them on the left side, and the ureter, the spermatic or ovarian, and the renal and colic vessels on each side. The external iliac artery lies medial to the psoas major in the pelvis, and beyond the inguinal (Poupart's) ligament the femoral artery lies ventral to it. The lumbar plexus arises between its origins from the vertebral bodies and discs and those from the transverse processes. The nerves springing from the lumbar plexus take courses subject to much individual variation through the muscle on the way to their destinations. Fasciculi of the muscle may thus be separated by the femoral (anterior crural) nerve or other branches of the lumbar plexus. The iliacus muscle in the region of the pelvis is covered by retro-peritoneal fat. The psoas muscle crosses its medial margin and from between the two muscles the femoral nerve usually emerges to pass into the thigh above the iliacus. Beyond the inguinal ligament the iliacus lies in front of the capsule of the hip-joint and the straight tendon of the rectus femoris, and is crossed by the sartorius."

PATHOLOGY

It is quite obvious that, with all these important organs, blood vessels and nerves lying in such close relationship, one would expect an interplay of any pathological influence between the psoas and the organs it contacts and equally between the psoas and the spine. Except for the tracking of a psoas abscess – the pathology of which makes its diagnosis obvious – any reference (other than those quoted) to pathological conditions affecting, or arising from, the psoas is rarely found in medical literature.

In osteopathic practice, however, we persistently find evidence of the effects of systemic toxaemias upon the muscle tone and also a more direct, low-grade, inflammatory reaction from visceral or organic diesase. The muscle loses its power of relaxation and becomes chronically contracted. If this continues to the extent of circulatory impairment, the muscle fibres commence to atrophy. These changes in the muscle irritate the embedded lumbar plexus and, due to the local circulatory and lymphatic congestion, we get a low-back pain, without doubt of visceral origin.

MUSCLE ACTION

Now, as regards the action of these most important muscles, there is such a diversity of opinion among text-books and medical authorities that one is almost tempted to disregard them altogether, especially as they are mainly based upon the dissection of the cadaver and not upon the study of the living body. Let us examine a few of these opinions and then compare them with those formed by such osteopaths as have attempted a close analysis of the muscle work in situ.

Sorbotta-McMurrich on the function of the psoas simply state that "its action is to flex the thigh, to inwardly rotate and to aid adduction."

Davis says its action equals "flexion of thigh and if the hip is outwardly rotated it acts as a weak internal rotator and from the normal position of the hip the psoas aids in external rotation."

Bowen and McKenzie have this to say "the angle of the pull across the pelvis edge is fairly favourable for flexing the hip, in spite of the fact that the origin of the muscle is so far to the rear of its insertion. It is, however, apparent that leverage improves as the limb is raised."

Duchenne admitted the normal action was difficult to isolate and in fact he was unable to do so with the exception of flexion of the hip.

Sir Colin McKenzie, probably the best medical authority gives its action as "flexion of hip and with knees extended flexion of trunk on the hips."

Morris, as well-known as Gray's Anatomy, says "The ilio-psoas is a powerful flexor of the thigh and the hip and a weak internal rotator. It also serves to flex the lumbar region of the spine."

McGregor, who simply states that it flexes the thigh and is a rotator of the femur, in his *'Synopsis of Surgical Anatomy'* sums up exceedingly well the vagueness surrounding the function of these muscles by quoting Professor Wright's explanation of Cunningham's description of the psoas muscle. He – (Professor Wright) says "Cunningham said it was a medial rotator of the femur until the axis of rotation of the femur became medial to the long axis of the psoas, when it became a lateral rotator. Professor

Wright used to repeat this twice, and seeing the look of misery on his students' faces, said, 'Well, if you don't understand it, just tell the examiner what I have told you'."

Amusing, you may say, but nevertheless true, and it would appear that while the majority of opinions are in accord in stating that flexion of the hip is one action, they are at variance as to whether psoas is an internal or external rotator. Flexion of the spine is mentioned only by one or two writers and unilateral side-bending not at all, except by osteopathic authorities.

We must, therefore, turn to H.H. Fryette, the osteopath in California, for fuller evidence of the living muscle in action. He describes the action of the psoas:

(a) as a flexor of the trunk on the thighs,
(b) as a flexor of the hip joint after the rectus femoris has accomplished about 10 degrees of flexion,
(c) as an external rotator of the hip, and
(d) as side-flexor of the spine if acting unilaterally.

In reference to (b), he explains that owing to the insertion of the psoas muscle into the lesser trochanter of the femur, this being posterior to the ilio-pectineal line, it is, in his opinion, impossible for this muscle to flex the hip from the standing position until the rectus femoris has first flexed the hip to roughly 10 degrees. This is probably what Bowen and Mackenzie mean in stating as quoted above, that "it is, however, apparent that the leverage" (in hip flexion) "improves as the limb is raised." It is possible, although rather vaguely expressed, that Cunningham is also of this opinion. Not mentioned by other writers, (d) is probably the most important of all from a mechanical and pathological point of view.

J.M. Littlejohn, W.A. Schwab in his clear and detailed series of articles on the low back in the Journal of the American Osteopathic Association – 1931-2-3, C.H. Downing and other osteopathic writers of renowned academic qualifications, have also given a great deal of time to the study of psoas malfunction and agree with Fryette's brilliant exposition on this subject.

PHYSIOLOGICAL MOVEMENTS

Our profession must of necessity be particularly interested in the body's mechanical adaptability to all forms of structural and organic malfunction. As osteopathic mechanical engineers, our philosophy of healing is based upon the repair of the human mechanism by adjustment of tissue to tissue, organ to organ and structure to structure. Again, we are here indebted to H.H. Fryette for his close analysis of R.W. Lovett's findings on spinal movements, his realisation of Lovett's mistakes and his presentation to the profession of a scientific thesis on the

'Physiological Movements of the Spine' upon which all osteopathic manipulative technique must be based, if we are to demand recognition alongside other allied scientific bodies, and his description of the mechanical reaction of the lumbar region in psoas dysfunction is classical. So to Fryette must be given the credit for a full and close study of the living muscle in action and its intimate relations to body mechanics.

There is no doubt that when the lumbar region is involved in psoas malfunction, the bodies of the vertebrae react in much the same way as they do in any form of mechanical disturbance – that is to say – given a unilateral psoas fibrositis, with the lumbar spine in normal easy flexion, the vertebral bodies will eventually sidebend toward that side by the pull on the antero-lateral attachments and those on the transverse processes, and will rotate to the opposite side – towards the convexity (flexion-sidebending-rotation). The greater the fibrotic contracture and consequent pull, the greater the amount of both sidebending and rotation. Given a bi-lateral psoas fibrositis, this would tend to pull the lumbar spine into flexion, except possibly the lower lumbar where the tendency would be toward extension, and a physiological locking would ensue and if, as is usually found, there is increased tension of one side more than the other, the bodies of the vertebrae would sidebend to the stronger pull, but would in this case tend to rotate toward the concavity (extension-rotation-sidebending).

W.A. Schwab observes that "unilateral psoas fibrositis either acute or chronic, exerting appreciable traction upon the lumbar region, produces with few exceptions a lateral shifting of the lumbar segments toward the same side. There is usually a lumbar curve with the convexity upon the involved psoas side. A concavity on the involved side occurs rather exceptionally when the upper lateral psoas fibres are involved. The typical condition just described, not the exceptional one, represents a pathological entity calling for definite treatment procedure to remove the causative factor of lumbar maladjustment.

In the case of bilateral psoas fibrositis the lumbar region may be laterally flexed to either side but it is usally convex to the side exhibiting the greatest tension. This bilateral involvement, together with the unilateral condition before described, more nearly approaches the condition of a true primary psoas fibrositis."

PRIMARY AND SECONDARY CONDITIONS

This clearly points out the difference in the reaction of spinal mechanics to a PRIMARY and a SECONDARY psoas fibrositis, and indicates how carefully the history must be taken into account and the delicacy as well as the thoroughness required in the initial examination. Personally, though my experience is, in comparison, limited, my findings of the mechanical reactions in the lumbar region accord with these opinions, although I would venture to say that the lateral shift of the lumbar area to one side or another is the initial prerogative of the gravely acute primary case (owing to the tremendous ease with which this exceedingly flexible area can give way passively in a lateral direction), rather than the established one actively bearing weight in the erect positon, and the mechanical end result conforms to the action of the rule, as laid down in Fryette's *'Physiological Movements of the Spine'*, rather the exception, as the amount and direction of rotation ultimately decides the mechanical pathway that has to be retraced before a subsequent permanent cure can be obtained, all other pathologies being equally dealt with.

It has been stated that when a fact contradicts a theory, the theory must go, and I think if treatment based on the interpretations of these authorities produces results, we should be prepared to interpret these results as facts. I suggest this statement is eminently applicable to the many and varied theories hitherto held in reference to the function of the psoas muscle and the treatment of its affections.

DIAGNOSIS

The diagnosis of these conditions is exceptionally interesting to the earnest physician. There is a typical and definite posture associated with these psoas conditions. The patient shows a pronounced tendency to keep the trunk in flexion, buckled as it were, from the point of the lesion and toward the involved side if unilateral; there is a FIXED and CAREFUL walk and, in the acute case, if the patient is left standing for long, the trunk flexion is increased, the knee of that side bent, and the foot turned outward.

The patient suffering an acute attack is extremely wary of being even touched and will certainly resist strongly all but the most delicate manipulative measure. Obliteration of the normal lumbar curve in an acute "lumbago", coupled with the ability of the patient to increase trunk flexion without a further increase in pain, should lead one to suspect psoas malfunction as a possible cause of the attack, especially so if the pain is increased in ratio as the trunk attempts to regain the erect position. Exaggeration of the lumbar curve in an acute condition might suggest involvement of the lower fibres of the psoas.

In chronic cases, especially the bilateral, the posture has all the appearances of the flat-chested, fashionable "young man about town" – an apparent flexion of the trunk forward, plus the "drooping" shoulders, via the upper lumbar and lower dorsal on a rigid lower lumbar. If unilateral, there is, coupled with this forward flexion, side-bending to the involved side and a lateral shift of the pelvis.

At the sign of the slightest chill, the muscle goes into further contraction and exaggerates these postural findings and the history will be one of repeated attacks (probably every winter) of so-called lumbago where the only apparent "cure" has been rest in bed. This, the patient will invariably tell you, he discovered himself after trying every form of treatment without relief.

These chronic cases can usually fully flex and regain an apparent erect position without pain, but a careful examination will reveal all these gross movements taking place from the hip joints and any extension of the trunk is obtained at the expense of the dorsal region, while the whole of the lumbar area is held in rigid fixation.

Other interesting points in the diagnosis of these conditions are that the acute case will be unable to lie prone on the treatment table, in fact, he will probably refuse to do so, and any attempt to extend the legs on the trunk, either from the erect or prone position, will be automatically resisted and the pelvis and lumbar region will move only as a "one unit" mass.

The same resitance will be offered to all efforts to extend the trunk on the thighs. In the chronic case, especially during a sub-acute attack, his attempts to achieve the prone position sometimes appear rather ludicrous, his lumbar and pelvis remaining in a fixed convexity while he is carefully balanced on his hands and knees. This convexity decreases in ratio to the length of time it takes the anterior muscle mass to achieve the degree of relaxation possible in his particular case.

In direct contrast to nearly all other types of low back pain, the psoas patient is more comfortable sitting in a low easy chair with knees flexed or legs raised, and this positon, with its approximation of muscular attachments, is the one preferred by the patient when seeking ease. During the intervals between attacks, he can do most things required in everyday circumstances even to digging in the garden, driving a car, or sitting at a desk all day. In fact, nearly all present day (I nearly said civilised) occupations and popular sports, as well as the modern environment, demand that the body be partially flexed most all its life except, of course, in the totalitarian states where erectness of figure (usually gained by the complete elimination of the spinal curves) seems to be the sole object. Muscular strength may ensue as a result of the calisthenics demanded by these states, but I doubt very much the ability of the organic and nervous system to endure any prolonged strain.

However, to return, if and when the psoas patient achieves the prone position, examination to discover the amount of mobility present in an anterior direction will, in the very chronic cases, meet a resistance impossible to imagine short of bony ankylosis, lessening in ratio to that of deep muscular contraction in those cases showing a lesser degree of involvement. Any test in this direction on the acute case, other than the most gentle attempt, will result in a reflex muscular spasm rather startling to behold. In fact, no other condition demands such careful and delicate handling, if satisfactory results are to be obtained, than these affections of the psoas muscles.

Osteopathically, therefore, we must realise that these muscles must be affected in any disturbances of the lumber spine, pelvis and hip joints. Their action is in direct contrast to those powerful extensors, the gluteii muscles, and for this reason in all pathological affections of the psoas you will find a corresponding amount of wasting of the extensor groups. In all cases of lateral lumbar curvature, whatever the cause or the mechanical type, one should examine for the amount of psoas involvement. A so-called posterior innominate can be caused by a unilateral affection of this muscle just as easily as being a causative factor.

Although practically the whole of the lumbar segments contribute to the nerve supply, the chief source of supply to these muscles is derived from between L. 2-3. It will be found that a lesion exists here in practically every case and special attention as well as great care should be given this area in all treatment.

Fryette says "the spinal lesion ... at the second lumbar vertebra, where the principal nerve of the psoas arises from the spinal cord, but if the lesion is at the third or fourth lumbar vertebra, the lower part of the muscle is most involved. These cases can stand much straighter than when the lesion is in the second lumbar. If the mechanics of the psoas is kept in mind, the reason for this is readily understood."

It is believed that no other muscle in the body (other than perhaps, in the cervical area) is more receptive to local or general toxaemia than psoas, and every effort should be made to find and eliminate all possible foci of infection. A history of V.D. or any severe adbominal operation or organic disease should act as a warning for investigation as to a probable toxic absorption.

Palpation can be had in suitable cases via the abdominal wall and slightly below and beneath Poupart's ligament.

RADIOLOGICAL DIAGNOSIS

From a radiological point of view, diagnosis can be considerably aided and in an acute case of psoas involvement, radiographs should be taken both from the standing and supine positions and the patient should be allowed to retain his natural position.

In the supine position, if the patient is in great pain, the ilium on the side of the lesion may be drawn up, and the knee flexed beyond 10 degrees. This must therefore be allowed for in the interpretation of any plate which may show a considerable amount of "apparent" pelvic distortion. The plate may in fact simulate pelvic structural pathology of a gross nature. The main point and value of the X-ray, however, lies in the shadow of the muscle. The affected psoas will be seen as a slender bulging outline compared to the comparative straight outline of its normal fellow. This is not only due to contraction but also, indeed principally, to the oedema and engorgement of acute inflammation.

In a chronic case, there may be little difference in outline between the two muscles, but the shadow of the muscle will show striations throughout as well as being lighter on the affected side. This is evidence of the chronic fibrous thickening of the muscle which, by producing increased density of bulk, renders the X-ray penetration more difficult.

To summarise:

A case of acute psoas involvement will show a bulging and swollen outline due to the inflammatory engorgement.

A case of chronic psoas affection will not necessarily show swelling, but will show a variation in light and dark shadows due to differences in fibrotic density.

TREATMENT

The treatment of these cases requires, more than anything else, restraint on the part of the osteopath. The tendency is to go right ahead to mobilise the lumbar spine and stretch the psoas muscle. This, of course, is what is required, but the manner in which it is done marks the difference between success and dismal failure.

Approach to this patient should be that of delicacy and a profound realisation of the pathology involved, otherwise you have lost a patient and, what is more, osteopathy has lost a supporter.

In the acute case (all other pathologies being considered) the best results can be obtained by placing the patient on the table in a modified Sims position, with the convexity of the lumbar curve uppermost. This position, itself, puts the involved muscle on stretch tension enough to commence with. Add to this light but firm pressure on the convex side with the thumbs, outwards and downwards from spinous processes to transverse processes and towards the table, commencing from below-up, and you will soon produce a degree of relaxation and mobilisation, as well as considerable relief from pain, which should mark the end of the first treatment. Subsequent similar measures should be applied until the patient can easily adopt the prone position without discomfort. From this stage, pressure applied either with the hands or a Taplin mobilisor on the appropriate table, to the lumbar area, in rhythm with the patient's respiration and going deeper as relaxation is obtained, will produce the quickest soft tissue results and leave the patient in condition to receive any articular adjustments possible. Judicious use of the swinging leaf on the McManis table, with all its degrees of movement, can be of more than considerable help, especially in the initial stages of treatment.

The chronic case requires similar handling until the same state has been reached except that it is possible to assist these cases further by a manipulation – or series of manipulations – under anaesthesia, to overcome some of the adhesive contracture which is present in the deeper substance of the muscle, but no attempt of this nature should be made while any acute pain is in evidence. From a mechanical adjustment point of view, the best technique to employ is undoubtedly the two-man technique as developed by Hoover, Fryette, Schwab, and others, as this enables the operators to exert corrective tensions in all and any directions with the minimum of discomfort to the patient, and this is always desirable.

ACCESSORY EXERCISES

Last, but far from being the least important in the treatment of psoas affections, is the question of exercises to retain the stretch and elasticity of the muscle gained as a result of the corrections obtained. These must be graded in their application to the stage of relaxation possible without provoking reflex muscle spasm.

Hanging by the hands from a door or horizontal bar, allowing the body to sag dead weight with knees flexed and toes just touching the floor, is splendid for commencing exercise. I have some of my patients deliberately lie face downwards on a light feather mattress which "gives" from the centre, allowing the whole body to go into extension. These passive exercises are repeated as often as possible. The length of time must be left to the discretion of the patient, as they must always be done just short of the point where pain would occur on returning to the normal position. The strain of the exercises should be felt, but on no account must they be carried to any degree of actual pain.

The old army gymnastic exercise of "on the hands down" at the same time allowing the pelvis to droop towards the floor (which was always contrary to army regulations), is an excellent method of producing a passive stretch of the psoas.

Other exercises adopted and used by osteopathic authorities are as follows:
1. Lying on back with sacrum resting on edge of table. Allow one leg at a time to hang loosely over the side, completely relaxed – from two to three minutes from the beginning.
   (Table must be high enough to allow feet to clear the floor.)
2. Lying over the side of table with cushion under sacrum. Allow both legs to hand loosely, arms extended above head and touching table at back.
3. Lying face downwards, place hands on table and attempt to push trunk upward, keeping it relaxed and allowing body to sag. At the same time keep pelvis in touch with table.

(After doing this exercise for a week or two, allow pelvis to leave table, balancing on toes and hands and allowing the whole body to sink towards the table in as relaxed a manner as possible.)

4. Lying face downwards with affected leg stretched out on table, and other leg hanging over side with foot on floor. Attempt to raise trunk from table with hand, keeping affected leg straight out.

NOTE:

These are not active exercises, but designed for passive stretching of the muscles involved and must be undertaken with care. In the beginning do not prolong these exercises for more than two or three minutes at a time, otherwise pain will follow. Only increase time of stretching when there is no pain nor stiffness after returning to normal from stretching position.

In conclusion, let me state emphatically that freedom from pain and relief in walking does not constitute a cure of these conditions and it must be thoroughly explained to the patient that he should continue under treatment until such time as the maximum of mobility has been secured both in spine and muscle tissue. He should be encouraged to continue his exercises for an indefinite period, especially at the end of his daily work, or after anything involving strenuous use of the body, to counteract his "psoas tendency."

DIAGNOSIS AND TREATMENT OF THE LOW BACK

PRELIMINARY EXAMINATION

The patient is presented, fixed in a given position, acutely ill, apprehensive, scarcely daring to breath for fear of pain. Such a condition will not admit of elaborate and detailed examination, but there will be no unnecessary increase of pain if the patient is allowed to lie quietly in his position of rest, during a brief investigation into the causes of his distress.

Most predisposing factors are ignored by the patient. He is only concerned by the predominant symptom of pain, and in the absence of a history of gross trauma, will even deny the existence of an exciting factor. The original onset of pain is of the utmost importance, however, and the patient must be led back by means of careful questioning. The process of interogation must also be directed to discover any alteration in the general state of health, which might suggest a neurological lesion, metabolic change or a toxic background.

Our primary concern, however, is that of pain. From the undue stress and strain preceding the onset, and the sequence and distribution of the painful syndrome. Where peripheral pain is most severe, radicular origin is more probable. In those cases where back pain is predominant there is more likely to be an involvement of the musculo-skeletal system. In the presence of a radicular syndrome, coughing, sneezing, bending and lifting will aggravate the condition. The effect of exertion is to increase the intra-spinal pressure, and further irritate the nerve roots and their coverings.

Acute mechanical injury will usually give a history of sudden pain, with subsequent improvement. Pain of a dull aching nature which becomes gradually worse, irrespective of rest, activity, or treatment, is characteristic of malignancy of the spine.

Low back pain that is relieved by bed-rest suggests arthrodial lesions of the lower lumbar, or sacro-iliac articulations. Patients who complain of stiffness on rising in the morning, improve after movement and then suffer a return of pain as long as weight bearing continues, provide evidence of chronic spinal arthritis, or a low grade inflammation of the musculo-ligamentous system.

True sciatic neuritis of root origin will cause the patient to awake at night, and walk about to obtain relief. In the sitting position, the painful lower extremity is extended, and the weight is supported on the buttock which is not involved. Movement of the trunk will tend to increase root tension, either by direct compression, or torsion.

Apart from irritation created by exertion, positional change or postural imbalance, the patient will often trace out the site and pathway of pain as follows:

Pain localised over the groin and down the inner thigh usually indicates lesion of the symphysis pubis, or the acetabulum.

Pain referred to the medial aspect of the knee suggests a posterior lesion of the innominate.

Pain in the back and groin which apparently follows the line of the anterior crural nerve, might point to renal tract involvement, with a lesion area extending from 10 D-2 L.

Pain in the buttock and external aspect of the thigh (lateral cutaneous nerve), indicates pathology at 4-5 L. Where pain covers the whole of the lateral thigh, there is likely to be direct strain of the Tensor Fascia Lata.

Pain from the mid-buttock, and passing down the back of the thigh, lateral side of fore-limb, and over the dorsum of the foot, points to lesion at 5 L-1 S.

Finally, the examination should yield any details concerning a history of sore throats, severe chills, or infection arising from teeth, gall bladder or kidneys.

PHYSICAL EXAMINATION

Having assisted the patient to stand, we proceed to note his postural behaviour. If the patient stands perfectly still betraying apprehension lest he be touched, or make a false move, one is led to suspect sprain, or some deep pathology, to the point of an acute periostitis within a joint, such as the sacro-iliac articulation. The symptoms are extreme sensitiveness, accompanied by heat, swelling and oedema. On palpation there will be a circle of exquisite tenderness surrounding the area.

This condition differs from the typical sacro-iliac strain, where pain is induced at the extreme of movement when testing for mobility.

If the patient tends to lean towards the painful side there is probably some organic condition producing a reflex spasm of the Quadratus Lumborum group.

Leaning towards the unaffected side represents an attempt to relieve irritation due to the approximation of inflamed articular surfaces, ill balanced weight bearing, or some form of root pressure, which is secondary to disturbance of spinal mechanics, and the skeletal-muscular system.

A tendency to lean forward, and towards a hip joint which is slightly flexed, suggests an acute psoas spasm, resulting from low grade infection, abscess or direct trauma to the 2nd and 3rd lumbar vertebrae. Pain is located here along the branches of the lumbar plexus, lying within the substance of the muscle, and sometimes a referred pain to the sciatic nerve.

EXAMINATION OF THE SPINE

Key lesions are found in the upper lumbar area. Pain is localised to an area involving 3 to 5 vertebrae, and the group is central to a lateral curve. Here the primary movement is side-bending towards the concavity of the curve, with rotation into the high side, or convexity of the curve. This type of group lesion can represent gross disturbance by direct trauma to the bodies of the vertebrae, intervertebral discs and cartilages.

It is recognised as the primary FLEXION-SIDEBENDING-ROTATION type of altered spinal mechanics, and plays an important part in the differential diagnosis and the choice of treatment. In the absence of a group curvature, pain is often limited to the lower lumbar area. The lesion is usually localised to one articulation only, which does not move away from the mid-line, but represents a torsional strain, involving the articulating facets, ligaments and cartilages. It is the result of some violation of the permitted range of motion in the articulation, and occurs when the spine is taken out of the neutral position, into flexion or extension, with rotation and sidebending superimposed.

Under these conditions, the spine takes on the characteristics of a flexible rod, so that when further rotation and sidebending is attempted, there is an increased torsional movement, with rotation preceding the sidebending. This type of lesion is known as the EXTENSION-ROTATION-SIDEBENDING maladjustment of spinal mechanics, in which both rotation and sidebending occur in the direction of the concavity of the curve thus produced.

THEORY OF APPLIED TECHNIQUE

The diagnosis of the acute low back must take account of the degree of pathology present, as determined by visual examination, palpation, and the fundamental laws of the physiological movements of the spine, as they apply clinically to the patient in this area.

There are wide variations in the tissue changes. These may be more marked on one side of the spine than on the other, more superficial or more deep in acute or chronic lesions, and can exist in widely differing lesions, or can occur together in different parts of the same lesion. It is in the diversity of proportion, type and location of tissue change, which accounts for the diversification in position, tension and impaired freedom of movement.

These pathological changes enter into our consideration only insofar as the oedema and/or fibrosis influence the tensions and resistance of the periacticular structures; thus determining the degree of force, and the nature and frequency of treatment. The basis of osteopathic procedure is the recognition of the alteration in character of the soft tissues surrounding a joint, the bony malrelationship, and the variation in the physiological movement of the joint. In other words, all manipulation must be adapted to accord with the specific requirements of the lesion to which the technique is applied.

There has been much misunderstanding in manipulative technique, and much difficulty in the way of its development as a result of the statement that, Nature Tends Towards the Normal. Although this is true in a general way, it is not true in the sense that spinal lesions tend towards self adjustment when generalised forces are applied. According to the late Dr Carl McConnell, general treatment should only be given in the constitutional diseases; in the anaemias, or in complete ignorance of what is wrong with the patient.

Corrective force must be applied with extreme precision if the tissue resistance at the point of lesion is to be successfully overcome. Under any other conditions, the lesioned joint will resist reduction, even at the expense of trauma, or, at least, increased relaxation in adjacent articulations.

The anatomical position of the spinal joint is one in which all the tension-bearing structures are in equilibrium, and weight is evenly distributed in the "easy normal" or "neutral" position. The joints are relaxed, and the tissues are ready to respond to normal stress without undue resistance.

In the lesioned segment, however, the anatomical position cannot be secured because of the tension pathology, but a relative degree of relaxation can be gained by placing a joint in its position of maximum ease, thus reducing any contraction of the supporting structures, and providing an opportunity for the introduction of corrective forces into the joint, without any increase of muscular or ligamentous resistance.

With the patient in the prepared position, mild traction is applied as far as the fixed point together with physiological or anatomical locking. The problem in technique is the careful control of this process, to create a lever for the operation of correction as far as the lesion point, without travelling into it, or beyond it. In attempting to accomplish accurate leverage in difficult cases, it is essential to separate the physiological movements, when locking the spine, to give the best results. That is to say, where a corrective force makes use of sidebending, there must always be an element of rotation, and vise versa, together with flexion and/or extension.

Having established the lesion point, and focussed the leverages via the physiological movements, the operator must exercise his tension sense in order to discover what is going on in the joint, and let this determine the degree and angle of force to be used in correction.

THE TECHNIQUE OF TREATMENT

In the management of the patient suffering from acute low back pain, rest is of primary importance. In some cases rest in bed is essential, in others physiological rest induced by restricted activity and some form of temporary support, such as adhesive tape, or by any other means available. The osteopathic treatment in this early stage, is directed to relax the irritated tissues to afford the patient rapid relief. It is important to remember that, in giving palliative treatment great care must be exercised to stop the treatment immediately there is evidence of change in the spasm, or tonicity, of the muscles and ligaments involved, or a palpable change in temperature.

The timing of treatment depends on the patient's reaction, and local conditions. Severe cases may have a return of increased tonicity in 5 to 6 hours, and two treatments per day will then be necessary. More usually, however, daily treatment is sufficient. Every endeavour should be made to get the patient on his feet as soon as possible, but we must remember that all treatment in the really acute case, whether active or passive, must be directed to reduce inflammation.

Having placed the patient in the supine position, and slightly elevated the legs, the operator stands at the foot of the table facing the patient, and gripping the ankles in his own axillae, and with the arms crossed, grasps the patient's right leg above the ankle with the right hand, and the left leg in a like manner with the left hand. The operator's body can then be used at will, to offer mild alternating traction and release, each for a period of about 5 seconds, taking care that the patient suffers no inconvenience. The whole process can be completed in 5 minutes, and is a valuable preparation for corrective treatment.

In those cases having a group convexity in the upper lumbar area, accompanied by excessive muscular tonicity on that side, and muscular contraction on the concave side, there is limited flexion and extension of the trunk in this area, and the usual tests for sidebending and rotation will indicate the lesion at the apex of the convex curve. Attempted movement in the direction of ultimate correction will cause a mild spasm of pain, whilst movement in the direction of exaggeration will be free from discomfort.

The patient should then be placed in the Sims position, lying on the concave side, the pelvis near to the edge of the table and the knees flexed. The first maneouvre is designed simply to de-rotate the vertebra in lesion, and for this purpose, the operator stands at the back of the patient, and placing his reinforced thumbs over the prominent transverse process on the convex side, applies pressure rhythmically with the patient's exhalation, downwards and cauldalwards.

The primary movement in this type of lesion is that of sidebending with secondary reverse rotation. In correction, it is necessary to preserve as neutral a course as possible, and reduce the sidebending in the direction of the concavity, as far as is compatible with the patient's pain. This can be done by lifting the patient's flexed legs at the ankles, thus tilting the pelvis towards the convex side of the curve, and then placing the upper leg behind the lower. Now apply thumb pressure over the transverse process in lesion on the convex side, rhythmically with exhalation, but short of any re-acting spasm, and yielding presure only slightly with inhalation, until the tissues begin to relax. Then, still keeping up the thumb pressure, grasp the upper knee with one hand and extend and abduct the leg. The result will be a reduction of the sidebending, coupled with the de-rotation.

Now instruct the patient to lie on the opposite side in the normal sidelying position, and the concave side uppermost. The upper leg is then taken into extension followed by adduction, gradually increasing the pressure until the tissues begin to release, and the convex curve tends to reverse. To complete, assist the patient on to his hands and knees, and encourage him to slowly sink back to his ankles, while lowering the trunk to the table and stretching the arms forward, in order to stretch the erector spinae muscles. Where taping is indicated, take care to cover from the gluteal muscles up as high as the 8th dorsal, with ample horizontal reinforcement across the lesion area.

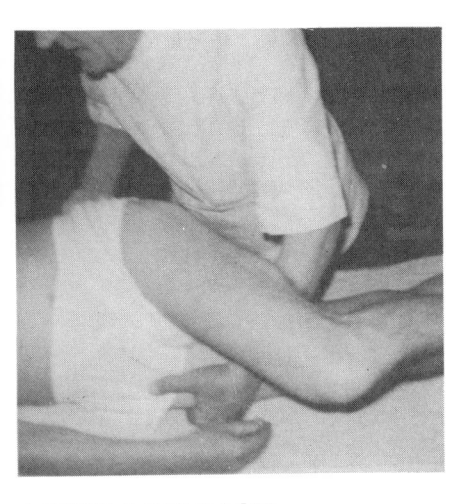

ACUTE LOW BACK
Turning the patient.
Convex side uppermost.

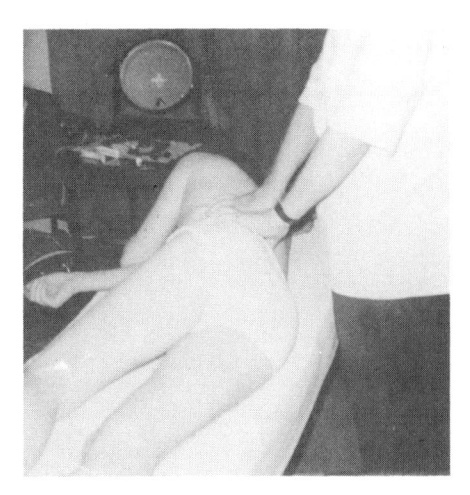

ACUTE LOW BACK
Relaxation of soft tissue.

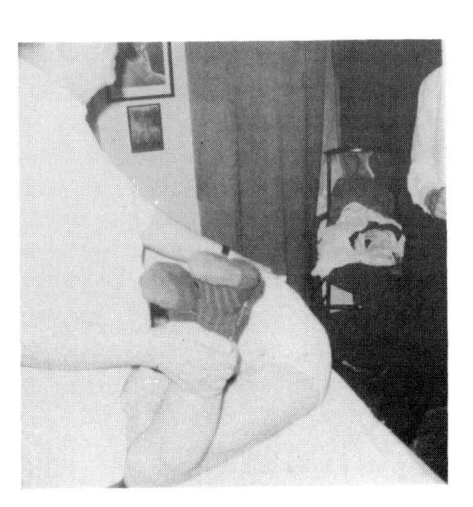

ACUTE LOW BACK
Long lever articulation.

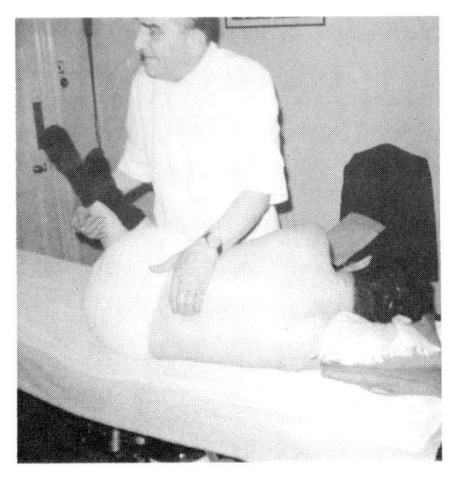

ACUTE LOW BACK
Long lever articulation.
(Reverse)

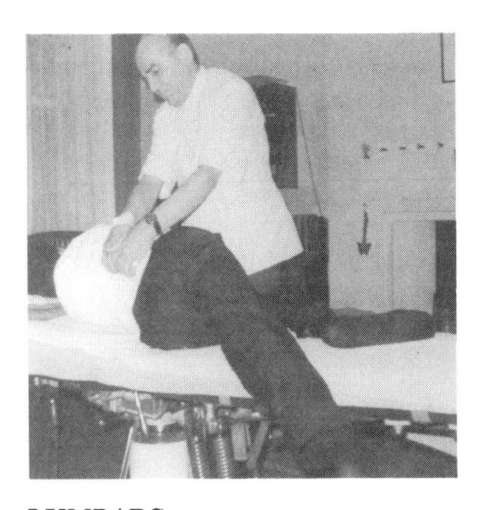

LUMBARS
De-rotation in acute. Convex side uppermost to start with.

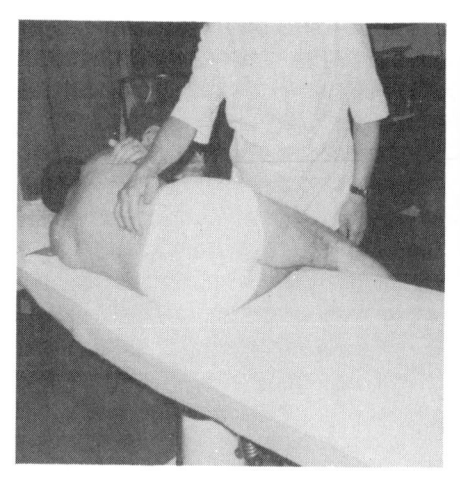

ACUTE LOW BACK
Concave side up.

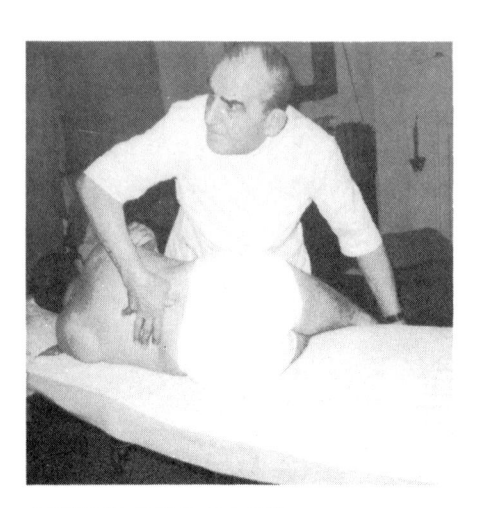

ACUTE LOW BACK
Using leg as long lever.

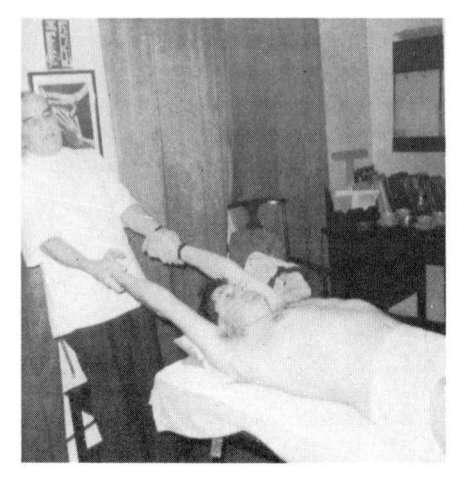

ACUTE LOW BACK
Traction and deep breathing.

TWO MAN TECHNIQUE

At the inaugural meeting of this Institute, held in 1954, the Chairman stressed the necessity of preserving and developing all techniques considered to be genuine osteopathy. In my view the two-man technique is genuine and original osteopathy and worthy of preservation. The two men most concerned in the origin of the technique as we know it today are H.H. Fryette and H.V. Hoover. It is less a matter of importance as to who was the first, but that it was adopted and is now practised by many of the leading osteopathic technicians throughout the profession. Nevertheless, there has been great danger of the technique becoming lost. I was particularly fortunate to have received separate instruction in this method from Drs Fryette and Chester Morris, and I was deeply impressed by the ease with which both operators accomplished their corrections. It was only after close questioning that I discovered they were paying greater attention to the minor movements and minor details of co-operation rather than to the gross movements as seen from the onlooker's point of view.

I can only hope by means of this paper and the demonstration to follow that these points can be made as clear to you as they were made to me. Previous attempts to explain and demonstrate the two-man technique at our post-graduate courses and conventions have not proved generally successful, but this may have been due to a lack of sufficient analysis in the presentation. However, the problem of survival of this particular technique, as I see it, presents two main difficulties. It calls for the close co-operation of two operators, and the work is laborious; yet it is only essential for one operator to know the principles upon which the technique is based, and any lay person such as wife, secretary or nurse, can be instructed in a few minutes to act as assistant. If strict attention is paid to the details of the part each one should play in the combined technique it is only a matter of time plus the experience of repetition to form a co-ordinated working team.

The heaviest work in performing this technique falls on the "pelvic operator" in the act of lifting the patient's knees from the initial position. Should the patient offer a slight resistance the weight is increased tenfold and there is undoubtedly a risk of severe strain to the operator's back if he is not already fixed in position. In order to avoid this danger the assistant operator is instructed to elevate and support the patient's knees until the pelvic operator can effectively grasp them without flexing his trunk.

Most specific work in osteopathic practice comes under the heading of fixed point technique. That is to say correction of the vertebra in lesion is accomplished by reversal of the mechanics of production round a point which is fixed by gravital stress, or physiological or mechanical locking. In contrast with this, two-man technique is based on a double contact designed mainly to producce simultaneous rotation of the two vertebrae involved, in opposite directions. Sidebending is introduced by the position in which the patient is placed plus the direction of the traction or torsion under the control of the operators. The basic principle of this technique is such that it may be applied to any type of inter-vertebral joint strain found in the lumbar area where there is malposition or immobility, giving rise to limitation of rotation and sidebending. The corrective leverages employed consist almost entirely of rotation and counter-rotation.

Irrespective of the type of lesion diagnosed, the patient is placed in the "Sims position" on that side towards which the spinous process of the vertebra in lesion is pointing: e.g., in the case of an extension-rotation-sidebending lesion to the right of the 4th on the 5th lumbar, the spinous process will be pointing to the left and the patient is placed in the left side "Sims position". In other words, the initial position is such that the transverse process of the lesioned vertebra which is posterior is uppermost, whether it is rotated posterior-inferior or posterior-superior.

If it can be assumed, then, that lesion of the 4th and 5th lumbar as described above, is present, the patient is placed on the left side and the left arm is allowed to drop over the back edge of the table. The knees are flexed and the pelvis is moved backwards to the edge of the table. The right arm is rested in a convenient position towards the top right-hand corner of the table.

Having thus completed the diagnosis and prepared the patient for correction, it is essential to decide on the choice of position of the number one man from which the operation is controlled. The designation of No. 1 and No. 2 man is not entirely satisfactory and I prefer the terms, "Spine or Trunk Operator", and "Pelvic Operator". According to Fryette the trunk operator should control the correction, while Chester Morris, on the other hand, preferred that the pelvic operator should assume control. It is of interest, perhaps, to quote briefly from my original notes recorded at the end of a day's work with Fryette. "He says that the trunk man controls the correction and he makes sure he does this part, mainly, I think, because the knee/pelvic part is heavy going and he even admits this. He seems to control the lesion by placing the pisiform side of his hand over the transverse process and pressing over the lumbar from below upwards, while holding the extended arm and wrist. Whereas Chester Morris prefers the fingers curled round the table side of the spinous processes while his forearm fits snugly round the waist line." In retrospect I think that the hold used by Chester Morris would provide a more rigid and localised tension-locking for the lumbar corrections, but Fryette's method is probably better for corrections of the pelvis.

With all these details confirmed the pelvic operator takes up his position behind the patient and opposite the pelvis. He then places his proximal knee firmly on the table close behind the flexed knees of the patient. From his position on the opposite side of the table the trunk operator raises the patient's knees about 10 degrees from the table, at which level the extended hand and arm of the pelvic operator is at the best mechanical advantage to grip and sustain the weight of the lower limbs. The trunk operator now grips the patient's right wrist with his right hand and, leaning over the patient, approximates his chest and shoulder to the postero-lateral side of the patient's thorax. The immobilisation of the upper part of the patient's body is thus secured by the operator's own weight, which may be usefully reinforced by carrying the patient's right arm downwards and outwards into full extension.

At this stage the pelvic operator's left thumb is braced over the spinous process of the 5th lumber vertebra and the trunk operator curls the 2nd and 3rd fingers of his left hand round the spinous process of the 4th lumbar. Both operators then slightly yield or exaggerate their respective levers until an optimum tension is engaged at the point of lesion. The double movements of rotation and counter-rotation are then made simultaneously at a given signal from the controlling operator, which consist of a sharp tug given under the spinous process of the 4th lumbar vertebra with a rapid thrust delivered in a downwards direction over the spinous process of the 5th lumbar.

This technique is of value in the treatment of both the flexion-sidebending-rotation, and the extension-rotation-sidebending types of lesion, and may be successfully applied to the whole of the lumbar area. In the flexion-sidebending-rotation type the "pisiform transverse process" contact is to be preferred, in which case the patient's knee flexion is increased in order that a rotation may be effected in conjunction with the pelvis, that is nearer the apex of the convex lumbar curve. With the extension-rotation-sidebending type, however, the curled fingers round the spinous process will give a better control, and here the knee/pelvic rotation is given a slightly more extended position. If properly executed these controls will take care of any sidebending which may be present in the lesion.

PELVIC TECHNIQUE

At this point I would like to digress for a moment to discuss one or two factors with reference to the mechanics of the pelvis. It has often been said that "you cannot have it both ways" but this two-man technique is not without interest in that equal results can be obtained whether we think in terms of movement of the ilium round a central axis at the second sacral segment, or of rotation round the upper or lower poles of the sacro-iliac articulation with all the resultant changes in the axes of movement. It will be an advantage, therefore, to avoid all complicated or controversial theories of pelvic mechanics for the time being. At least we can agree that if a lesion is produced within the pelvic ring under the conditions of weightbearing, it will not long remain an individual lesion, and that compensation will rapidly take place within the pelvic ring as well as above and below it.

In the attempt to preserve the equilibrium, the sacrum and/or the unaffected ilium will begin to accommodate to the primary lesion strain, which means that if one innominate moves in lesion the other will move in the opposite direction with a resultant torsional strain of the sacrum, e.g., the up-anterior or posterior lesion of the ilium may also be described as an anterior sacrum on the same side. Conversely, the up-posterior or anterior lesion of the ilium can be alternatively named a posterior sacrum on that side. Both types of lesion on either side will respond to this type of treatment. Whatever our individual theories might be concerning the mechanics of lesion production in this area there is no doubt that the two-man technique is particularly suitable for correction in that both aspects of the sacro-iliac lesion are placed under control at one and the same time.

If it can be assumed that we have a lesion of the pelvis in which compensation has taken place, i.e., an up-anterior or posterior ilium on the left, and an up-posterior or anterior ilium on the right, the patient is placed on his left side in the "Sims position" with a view to the correction of the left ilio-sacral articulation. The trunk operator then takes up his position as for the lumbar correction except that his proximal hand (left) is placed over the lumbo-sacral junction in a manner that will bring maximum effort to bear on the left sacral articulation. The fingers are locked round the 5th lumbar and the 1st sacral spinous processes and the heel of the hand exerts pressure over the erector spinae mass covering the uppermost transverse processes. The chest contact and the right hand traction are then brought into play and the rotation is carried throughout the entire spine into the sacro-iliac articulation on the table side.

The position of the pelvic operator is also similar to that of the lumbar correction but in this case his flexed right knee is placed as close as possible to the patient's pelvis, and his left thumb is directed over, and slightly above the posterior-spine of the patient's left ilium. Both operators now "tease for tension" as it were until maximum stress is brought to bear on the articulation in lesion, and the correction is made by a slight exaggeration of these movements in combination with a sharp thrust from the pelvic operator's thumb.

In the treatment of the opposite side the patient's position is reversed and the "Sims position" is again adopted. The technique is similar except for three minor but important changes; (1) The patient's knees are flexed nearer to the patient's abdomen. (2) The thrust, as applied by the pelvic operator, is delivered over the posterior inferior spine of the right ilium or the lower part of the posterior superior spine. (3) The trunk operator must apply a firm pressure over the base of the sacrum in order to tip the apex of the sacrum in a posterior direction thus meeting halfway the forward and downward movement of the ilium as initiated by the pelvic operator.

It must be remembered that "A manipulation must consist of a force acting against a resistance in a certain direction at a given speed, and as this resistance constantly varies, so must all factors concerned in the correction be capable of infinite variation". Although this statement is true of all specific technique it applies more particularly to the two-man technique, and especially in the treatment of the pelvis. Therefore, it is essential to make sure that all leverages are carefully co-ordinated up to the point of maximum tension before the final adjustment is attempted.

In my opinion this "rotary two-man technique" is most useful in the treatment of lesions involving pregnancy, and in all manipulations of the low back and pelvis given under anaesthesia. It is also the technique par excellence for the ballet dancer, the acrobat and all the hypermobile types of back. It may equally well be applied to the chronic fibrotic lesion, and the short, bulky muscular type of patient.

It now only remains to consider, very briefly, the "Two-man Tug Technique". As the title suggests this is a method which is based on the principle of a straight pull without any element of rotation. In preparing the patient for correction the ordinary side-lying position is adopted and the lesioned ilium is placed uppermost from the table. The arms are flexed at the elbows and rested close to the anterior thorax: this serves to provide the trunk operator with an improved hold and avoids the risk of injury to the patient.

This technique is the method of choice in the treatment of that most difficult lesion the primary up-posterior, or anterior innominate. Clinically we know that the subjective symptomatology produced by this type of lesion is located both laterally and below the posterior superior spine, and that this is the area where the ligamentous pathology is most evident. It is for these reasons that the tension should be centred here before the tug is applied.

Therefore assuming a lesion of the right ilium the patient is placed in the left lying position. Standing at the back of the patient the trunk man places his flexed left arm over the patient's flexed arms, and approximates the lateral side of his body to the patient's chest. The operator is now in a favourable position to control, or hold in fixation, the patient's right innominate and this can be done most conveniently by placing the left hand over the iliac crest with the palm over the anterior superior spine, while the palmar surface of the right hand is fitted firmly and snugly over and below the posterior superior spine.

At this stage in the preparation the "Tug Operator" assumes his position on the opposite side of the table and takes up the patient's right leg. The knee is flexed with the right hand supporting the tibial head, and the left hand supporting the ankle. The leg is then gently flexed until the trunk operator signals that muscular and ligamentous tension is accumulating under his right hand. At this point, and without any change of angle, the leg is fully extended, and from this position is slowly abducted and adducted until the trunk operator again signals a reaction under his right hand, which, for the want of anything better may be described as a "gapping strain" at the articulation.

The successful completion of the "Tug Technique" demands a degree of balanced co-operation which is even more important than in the rotatory method. In the majority of cases it is necessary to induce relaxation in the patient by means of deep regular breathing, or by gently moving the extended leg, and when sufficient relaxation hs been gained the leg is then externally rotated and placed under mild, but sustained and increasing traction. The correction is finally made by a slight but sharp tug which is applied *without releasing* the traction. The trunk operator is not required to thrust but merely to guide along the plane of the articulation, although he should be aware of movement in the sacro-iliac joint.

I have been at pains to present this two-man technique in some detail because I feel that the benefits of the work of Fryette and Hoover in this field should not be lost to the profession. Although it is difficult to describe and demands care in application, the technique is capable of gaining results where other methods have failed. If I may end on a personal note it is worth recalling that on the occasion of Dr Fryette's visit to this Institute last year he remarked that, having spent a lifetime in teaching osteopathy, he considered the two-man technique to be his major contribution to the growth and development of osteopathy, and that he would be content to be remembered for his pioneer work in the discovery of this technique alone.

DIAGNOSIS AND TREATMENT OF THE LOWER DORSAL SPINE

The subject of our demonstration is the diagnosis and treatment of lesions of the lower dorsal spine, but some introduction is necessary in the form of a short general discussion of the area from the viewpoint of physiological movements, lesion tendencies and symptomatology in terms of the nerve connections of the area.

First a definition. We have included in the lower dorsal area all segments from D5 - D12 inclusive. We have done so because this corresponds to the so called splanchnic area, associated with the greater, lesser and least splanchnic nerves, in spite of the fact that it includes two thirds of the dorsal area. And it must be stressed that from the point of view of the physiological movements of the spine this is a purely arbitrary grouping, since these movements are by no means constant throughout the area.

The chief movements in the thoracic spine are flexion and extension, but even these are strictly limited in the upper segments, and only become free in the lower three. Flexion is the less restricted of the two movements, since the angle of the facets and the separation of the ribs posteriorly aid flexion more than extension. In the lower three segments both movements are relatively free.

The compound movements of extension-rotation-sidebending and flexion-sidebending-rotation are again limited in the upper segments by the approximation of the ribs. In extension, any degree of sidebending must be preceded by rotation to carry the upper ribs posteriorly to avoid locking and impingement on the lower ribs. In easy normal, or flexion, sidebending is followed by rotation to the convexity in the manner which is familiar in the production of scoliosis. In the lower segments both these compound movements are free, with the sidbending component predominating.

The extreme lower limit of our area, the dorsolumbar junction, is a transition area, in which the angle of the facets changes abruptly from the coronal plane of the dorsal area to the sagittal plane of the lumbar. The type of movement permitted between the 11th and 12th dorsal vertebrae and that permitted between the 12th dorsal and 1st lumbar is different, and the possibilty of lesioning at this level is correspondingly increased.

Rib movements are of two main kinds, the so called bucket-handle and pump handle movements. In the former the axis of motion is a line drawn from the costo-sternal articulation to a point between the costo transverse and costo vertebral articulation; and movement of a rib, about this axis raises or lowers the shaft of the rib, and increases or decrease the transverse diameter of the thorax. In the pump handle movement the axis is drawn between the costo transverse and costo vertebral articulation and the neck of the rib rotates on its long axis, thus raising or lowering the sternal end of the rib and increasing or decreasing the anterior posterior diameter of the thorax. These two movements are normally combined in a compound movement containing both components. In the lower two floating ribs this does not apply since the anterior ends are free, and movement here, although slight, takes place in all directions, and is termed enarthrodial.

The nerve connections of the lower dorsal area include the greater, lesser and least splanchinic nerves which supply the intestinal tract from the stomach to the transverse colon, the liver, pancreas, kidneys and adrenals, and most of the structures of the urogenital system. These are the pre and post ganglionic fibres of the sympathetic system, travelling via the coeliac and superior mesenteric ganglia.

In addition there are the intercostal nerves supplying the segmentally related somatic structures, and carrying also the vaso-motor, pilo-motor and sudo-motor nerves. Finally there is the nerve supply to the diaphragm, coming partly from the phrenics and partly from the lower six intercostals, the pleural and peritoneal covering being supplied by the vagus and sympathetics.

The importance of a properly functioning diaphragm can hardly be overestimated, and its influence upon the thoracic and abdominal viscera is profound. The splanchnic nerves and the ganglionated chain pass through the crura of the diaphragm, and the coeliac ganglia lie on the surface of the crura. The integrity of the lower dorsal spine and ribs is thus seen to be of great importance in the functioning of the diaphragm and through the latter in the functioning of neurologically related viscera.

Diagnosis and correction of lesions in the lower dorsal can hardly be reviewed without reference to changes taking place in areas above (mid and upper dorsal) and below (lumbar, lumbo-sacral and pelvis) and especially at the dorso lumbar, where the changeover from coronal to sagittal facets in the 12th dorsal – 1st lumbar poses its own particular problem.

This lower dorsal region accommodates itself very easily to strain in any other part of the body, particularly to postural imbalance and pelvic torsional imbalance. The transitional nature of this area must be involved in the strain of maintaining the erect position especially in a compensating manner following such conditions as Primary short leg, errors in locomotion, Psoas muscle contracture and even the simple individual Ilial lesion. The muscles of the back also play an important part in any disturbance of this area exclusive of the Erector spinae group, e.g. the Latissimus Dorsi arising from the crest of the ilium on its way to the upper extremity has attachments separately to the lower three ribs. The

Quadratus Lumborum, short and powerful, from Pelvis to 12th rib, represents tension strain in any lateral deviation of this area. In any review of this lower dorsal area, the last six ribs must be taken into consideration as apart from the costo-vertebral and costo-chondral articulations, we must recollect the crura of the diaphragm and its attachments to these six lower ribs as well as to the upper Lumbar Vertebrae.

Individual lesions certainly do occur in this region but in our experience mainly have to be sorted out from within some compensating curve which is either exaggerating a normal Kyphosis or a lateral curve shifted from the mid line of the spine.

These single lesions found here seem to exercise a lot more influence in disturbance of reflexes and of visceral functions than in other parts of the body; no doubt the lumbar enlargement of the spinal cord which commences at the 10th dorsal could account for the variations in vaso motor control and pain referred to areas remote from this lesioned region.

Diagnosis in this area should follow the pattern for diagnosis in any other part of the spine – siz. Visualisation–Palpation–Mobilisation tests. This area pays dividends when *visualised* in the standing position, trunk flexion and extension, and sitting and prone positions. Flexion and extension lesions practically stand out on their own, singly or collectively, and gross rotations are obvious. This should be followed by *Light Palpation* to determine changes in temperature painful or tender spots, deviation, gross or otherwise, of the spinous processes, tension of surrounding tissues, muscles and ligaments. Spasm in muscle is usually to be found on the side of vertebral rotation with tenderness to pressure; deep tenderness is more often located on the side to which the spinous process has moved. In the tests for *mobility*, one should bear in mind that movement in the direction of correction elicits more pain or resistance than movement in the direction of exaggeration; deep mobilisation pressure gradually applied with the patient in any position will also indicate the particular intersegmental articulations involved. We should also remark here that the physiological movements of the spine as described by Fryette should be strictly interpreted in dealing with this particular area. Leverages applied for diagnosis in this area are legion but it should be obvious that the ones that can be applied while leaving the hand or hands free for the delicate interpretation of tissue findings and mobility changes should be chosen where possible.

A point we think is insufficiently stressed in this area in relation to the art of technique, is the application of the Body Triangle. This triangle is represented by the operator's two arms with elbows flexed, and his body as the base of the triangle. The area under treatment is contained within the triangle and the rule is:

That all angles of the triangle should be approximated toward the centre, as represented by the lesioned area, to reduce the risk of strain to the patient and to the operator. The operator's body posture should be accommodated to the triangle throughout the execution of all techniques used in correction.

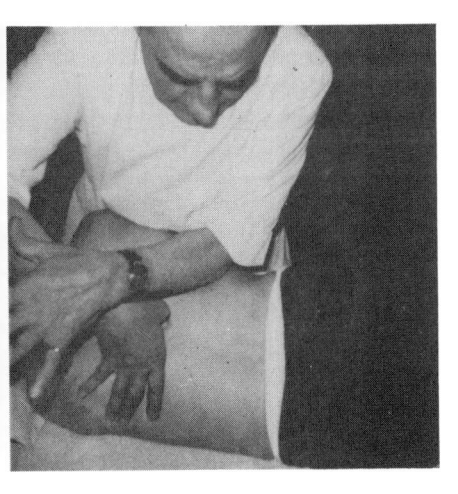

RIBS (lower)
Elbow thrust with stabilisation of
spinous process.

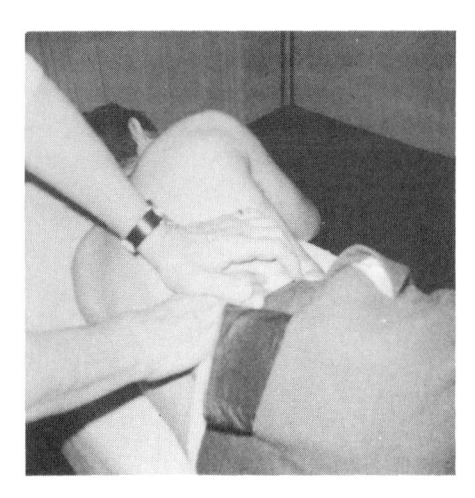

12th RIB
Thrust

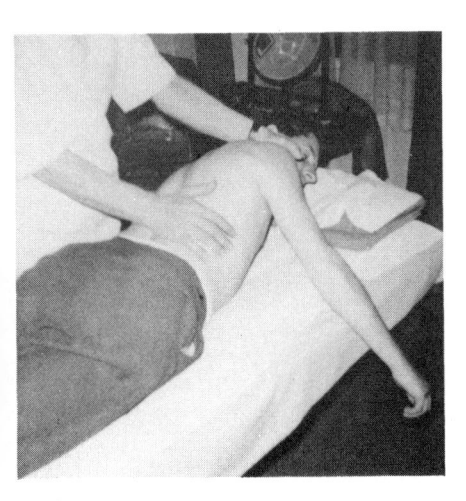

12th RIB
Long arm thrust.

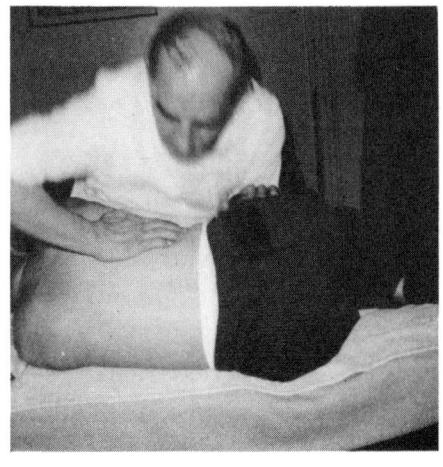

RIBS
Long arm thrust on angle of rib.

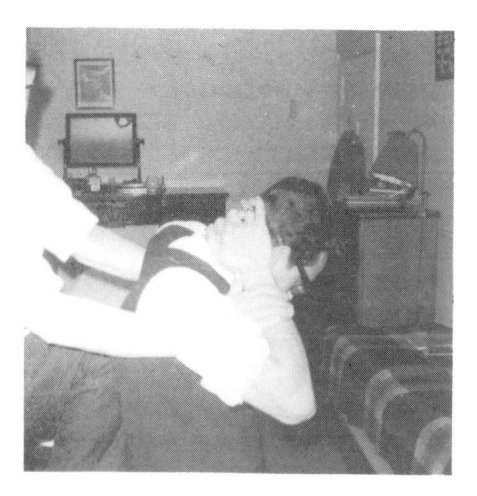

DORSALS
*Knee technique
(starting position).*

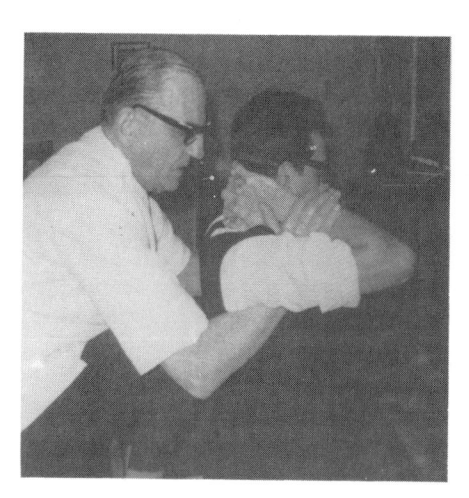

DORSALS
*Knee technique
(finishing position).*

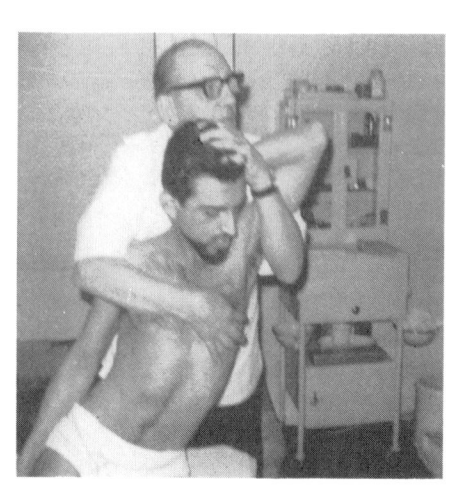

RIB ELEVATION
Sitting technique (1)

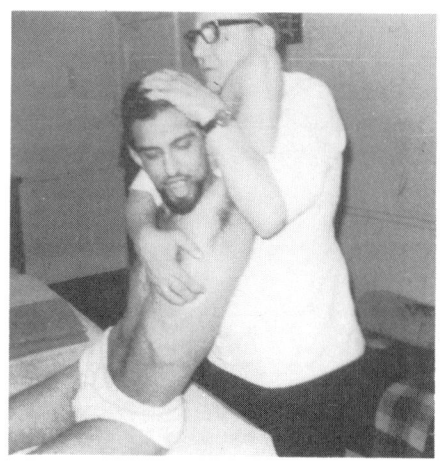

RIB ELEVATION
Sitting technique (2)

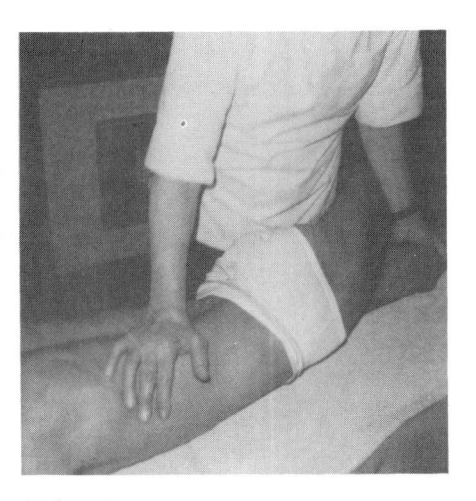

12th RIB
Long lever technique.

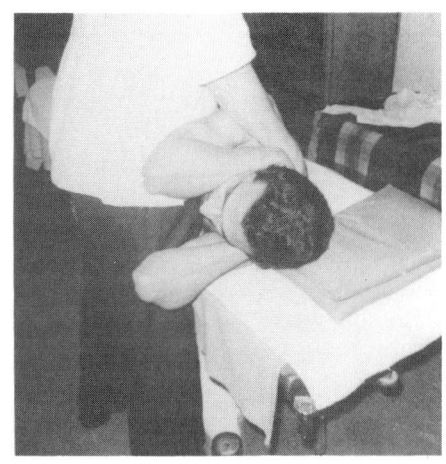

DORSALS (1)
Hands behind neck.
Elbow lever technique.
1) Arms 2) Location of lesion 3) Roll

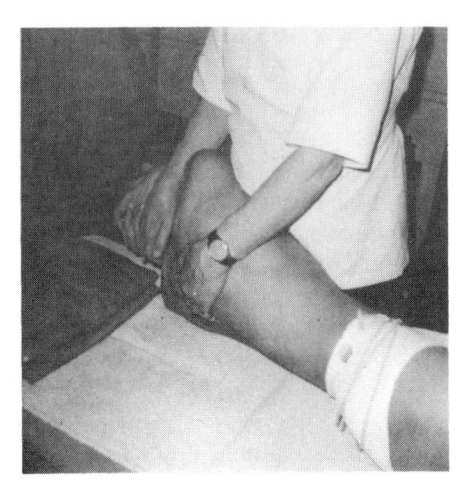

DORSALS (2)

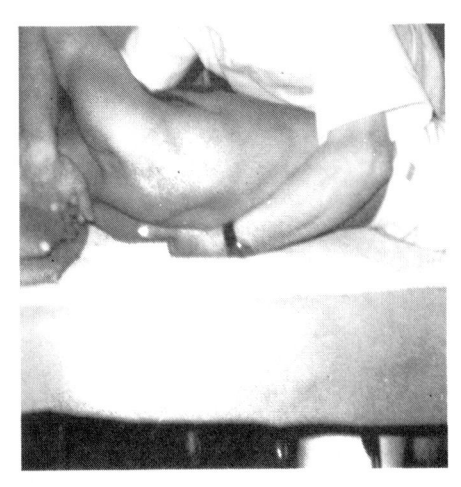

DORSALS (3)

THE OCCIPITO-ATLANTAL ARTICULATION

This is not an area that lends itself to an easy description so I propose to go straight in to a quote from H.V. Halliday's "Applied Anatomy of the Spine" on movements of this articulation.

Movement. "Impairment of movement is one of the first indications of lesion of this articulation. Palpation should be made carefully and correctly, taking every factor in the discussion of the joint into consideration. This articulation may be the primary seat of lesion, but may also be secondary and in all cases thorough examination of the entire spine should be made so as to determine the possibility of this articulation attempting to compensate for lesion below."

You will be thinking that this description applies to any other lesion anywhere in the spine, and of course, you are right. In fact, MacWilliams of Boston actually lists the lesions that are complementary to each other throughout the spine, the pelvis and the ribs, and his views are in the main accepted by the profession, although I daresay most of us are not so thorough in our detailed diagnosis, but I believe that "if you look you will find," and definitely so in this articulation.

However, I also feel that the occipito-atlantal articulation is very special in the lesion field, and with this in mind, and because I like to think that all Technique in Osteopathy should be taught alongside applied anatomy, I ventured to check up on a variety of text books on anatomy and applied anatomy to see what they had to say on this articulation. I found this very interesting, if only for the difference in the approach of each author on this articulation and the amount of information they considered it merited:

Gray, E.G.	was rather cold, complex and precise
Morris	also rather cold but occasionally human
Grant	essentially scientific
McGregor	very, very good precise reading
Beckwith	brilliant on pure mechanics
Guy	theoretetically marvellous, but you need to be almost a physicist to follow him
Downing	Osteopathically excellent, but too many mistakes (He says they occur at the printers)
Clark, M.E.	clinically logical and humane (Applied Anatomy)
MacLoughlin	first class arrangement – great detail (Anatomy in a nutshell)
Halliday	precise – concise for students (Applied Anatomy abbreviated to be carried around with one)

(The last six authors are osteopaths.)

I have chosen to use Dr M.E. Clark's description of this articulation for reasons that will become obvious as we go along. His method of presenting this area appeals to me in that he tells me something that is interesting with every other line, and brings a little humanity into a subject that is usually dealt with as dead anatomy. Dr Clark's book is one that is written by an osteopath for osteopaths, and should be in every osteopath's library despite its age (50 years?). (His *'Diseases of Women'* is equally good.)

This joint is variously described as Ginglymoid, Double Condylarthrosis, partial ball and socket, etc. Descriptions of the applied anatomy of this articulation more often than not commenced with the atlas, probably because it has 10 pairs of muscles attached to it from above and below, and, as a point of interest, in the technique of overall adjustment of this articulation it is as well to remember that the axis has 14 pairs of muscles attached to it.

Clark says "The atlas is the most peculiar of vertebrae. It is the uppermost of the vertebrae forming the spinal column and supports the head. For an object to be well supported, there must be little motion between the part supporting and the part supported. This is true of the atlas and occiput, the atlanto-occipital articulation being to all intents and purposes immovable, very little motion at least, taking place at this joint in movements of the head. On this account lesions of this articulation are rare as compared with other vertebral articulations, using the term lesion in its usually accepted meaning. In the better use of this term, that is including all affections of the articulation, especially sprains of the ligaments, a lesion of this articulation is quite common."

The atlas is peculiar in that the body is absent, it being supposedly usurped by the odontoid process of the axis. This is of interest since complete dislocations result in pressure on the spinal cord by the odontoid process from breaking of the transverse ligament, and paralysis of all parts below follows if pressure is constant and long continued. The absence of the body of the atlas makes it thinner, thus permitting of freer motion of the head of the spinal column, in accordance with the general rule that the smaller the vertebra the greater the arc of mobility.

The posterior spinous process, which is developed in all the other vertebrae, is absent, or, at least, poorly developed in the case of the atlas. There is a rudimentary process or tubercle that takes its place, and to which is attached the small posterior recti muscles. Ordinarily, it cannot be palpated even though the neck be in flexion, but in some cases it is possible to distinctly palpate it. If it can be palpated it denotes either (1) an abnormal development of the tubercle; (2) an anterior condition of the occiput on the atlas; or (3) a posterior condition of the atlas, the atlas and occiput being displaced posteriorly on the spinal column. The diagnosis is based on (1) great tenderness over and around the tubercle, and (2) disturbance of function of the articulations of the atlas. If there is no tenderness in or around the articulations of the atlas and the function is unimpaired, the prominence of this tubercle is not pathological but a peculiarity.

At the junction of the anterior arches is another tubercle. It is of interest in that the longus coli muscles and the anterior vertebral ligament are attached to it, hence in lesions of the atlas flexion of the head and neck may be impaired indirectly, by affecting these muscles through their nerve supply or attachment and directly, by derangement of the articular facets.

The superior articular facets are peculiar on account of their shape, size and the direction that they face. These facets are oval shaped, deeply concave from before backward, converge in front and incline obliquely inward. They are often indented in which cases they are divided into two unequal parts, thus lessening the mobility of the joint. They receive the condyles of the occipital bone, thus forming a rather secure articulation. On account of the depth of the concavity of the superior facets of the atlas and the prominent convexity of the occipital condyles, dislocation of this articulation either partial or complete is rare. Also the facets act as inclined planes, thus assisting spontaneous reduction if the condyles were forced slightly upward on the facets. By muscular contracture the occiput and atlas are approximated, this of itself lessening the mobility of the occipito-atlantal articulation. If, in addition, an inflammatory exudate is present from meningitis, influenza or other causes, mobility of this articulation is still further lessened. The principal movement of this joint is an antero-posterior one, thus permitting of a nodding movement of the head.

Another peculiarity is the fact that the articular facets of the atlas, like those of the axis, are anterior to the place of exit of the spinal nerves: the facets being posterior in all the other vertbrae.

There is a circular facet on the posterior surface of the anterior arch for articulation with the odontoid process of the axis. On account of this articulation a displacement of the atlas directly backwards is impossible unless it carries the axis with it.

The inferior facets are smaller and more nearly circular than the superior, but like them, concave. They face inwards and downwards and are more subject to abnormal movement than are the superior. This is because of the freedom of movement and the leverage exerted on it by the atlas and occiput.

The movements of the atlanto-occipital articulation are not very well marked: they consist principally of a rocking movement of the occipital condyles on the superior facets of the atlas. This has been described as of a ginglymoid character. Morris says: "There is also a slight amount of gliding movement, either directly lateral, the outer edge of one condyle sinking a little within the outer edge of the socket of the atlas, and that of the opposite condyle projecting to a corresponding degree. The head is thus tilted to one side, and it is even possible that the weight of the skull may be borne almost entirely on one joint, the articular surfaces of the other being thrown out of contact. (Lateral occiput). Or the movement may be obliquely lateral, when the lower side of the head will be a trifle in advance of the elevated side." (Oblique occiput).

The head is so poised on the superior articular surfaces of the atlas that it requires little muscular effort to keep it balanced. If the occiput or atlas become changed in position as a result of a subluxation, the balancing of the head becomes more difficult, that is, more muscular effort is required to keep the head in a normal position Since the cervical ligaments have little or nothing to do with the balancing of the head, and since the muscles connecting the head with the spinal column are the principal factors concerned in holding the head erect, it follows that any disorder of these muscles or the joint itself, will interfere with this function, that is, the head is drawn too far to one side or else the balance is lost so that it moves to and fro. Many of the cases characterised by a constant nodding movement of the head are due to some affliction of either the joint itself or the nervous mechanism moving the joint so that the muscles are constantly drawing the head out of balance, that is, it is drawn too far foward or backward in the attempts of the cervical muscles to keep it poised. This articulation should be checked in all cases of astigmatism, diplopia, strabismus, nystagmus, proptosis and ears with semi-circular canal imbalance. If the lesion exists for some time the irritation is not overcome by assuming the prone posture but as a rule the movement is decidely lessened in the worst cases and is stopped entirely in the mild cases. If prone posture is assumed for several hours as in sleep, the attempts of the muscles to balance the head cease. The above is the principal cause of nodding the head.

The first cervical nerves making their exit in relation with the atlas, pass along a groove over the posterior arch instead of through a foramen. This groove being occasionally converted into a foramen. The vertebral vessels also pass along with the first cervical nerve.

The transverse processes are unusually large and rough and extend farther outward than those of the other vertebrae. They are perforated by a foramen through which pass the vertebral vessels and vertebral plexus of nerves. Numerous muscles are attached to the transverse processes, in contractured conditions of which the position of the processes is changed. These processes are quite superficial, hence tender on pressure. Use is occassionally made of this fact in treating hysterical cases, pressure on the transverse processes producing such pain that the patient forgets about the other trouble. The direction and position of the processes vary in different individuals. Theoretically they should point directly outward and be midway between the angle of the jaw and the mastoid process. The position of the head is sometimes indicative, if not diagnostic, of a lesion of this articulation. If the chin is drawn in abnormally far, the chances are that the head sets too far back on the spinal column (posterior occiput) that is on the atlas; if the chin protrudes unusually far, the opposite condition exists. The sterno-mastoid muscles are put on a tension in the first, and relaxed in the second condition. (anterior occiput).

The ligaments binding the atlas to the occiput are arbitrarily divided into anterior occipito-atlantal, posterior occipito-atlantal, two capsular and two anterior oblique. They are band-like elastic and densely woven ligaments and, if not diseased, hold the superior facets of the atlas and the occipital condyles securely in apposition.

The anterior occipito-atlantal ligament is composed of very strong dense fibres; they radiate upward and slightly outward from the anterior arch to the anterior common, the capsular and the atlanto-axoidean ligaments.

The posterior occipito-atlantal ligament is incomplete on both sides for the passage of the vertebral vessels and the suboccipital nerve.

It extends from the upper part of the posterior arch of the atlas to the posterior border of the foramen magnum. It is not very strong, is not stretched very tightly and does not to a great extent limit motion. Being weaker than the anterior, extreme flexion is more likely to produce a serious effect than is extreme extension. Because of the greater strength of the anterior ligament, the front part of the articulation is held the more securely in place than is the posterior, thus the latter would respond to a force more quickly than the former. The capsules do not materially strengthen the joint since they are quite lax. They entirely surround and enclose the occipito-atlantal articulation. They are reinforced and strengthened by the anterior oblique ligaments.

These ligaments are affected in various ways by bony and muscular lesions of the neck. However, the principal effects are those of relaxation and contraction or shortening. If the lesion is irritative the ligaments are likely to become thickened less elastic and shorter, and thus draw the head quite firmly down on the atlas. In the anemic and malnourished, relaxation takes place with increased mobility.

The blood supply to these ligaments comes principally from the vertebral while a few twigs are given off by the ascending pharyngeal. The innervation is from the anterior division of the first cervical nerve. In subluxations of the occiput, these ligaments are injured, either torn or badly stretched. This results in a thickening of the ligaments and deposits around the injured part. These conditions interfere with the function of the joint, the blood-vessels, the nerves in relation, the muscles attached and the intervertebral foramina that is the space between the posterior arch of the atlas and the axis.

The brain has a pulsation in the direction where the resistance is least. This is seen best in babies before the fontanelles close. The diastole and systole of the brain are in part made possible in the unyielding box of the cranium by the ebb and flow of the cerebro-spinal fluid. Hill says: "The occipito-atlantal and other vertebral ligaments extend in cerebral diastole, and allow the fluid to escape from the cranial cavity, while in systole through the elasticity of these ligaments coming into play, it is driven back." This then is an important factor in the circulation of the brain. Lesions of the occipito-atlantal articulation affect the ligaments and thus interfere with their elasticity. Since in all vertebral lesions the ligaments in relation are always affected, the direct relation of spinal lesions, and especially cervical, to brain disorders, becomes the better understood. (The Still Hildreth Sanatorium for the mentally sick noted the frequency of lesions of this articulation and at the fourth dorsal. Many prominent osteopaths have confirmed these observations.)

The ligaments uniting the atlas to the axis are the anterior and posterior atlanto-axoidean, capsular and the atlanto-odontoid.

The muscles attached to the atlas are the recti capiti minores and laterales, longus colli, obliqui, splenius colli, levator anguli scapulae and the intertransversales. Most of these are attached to the transverse processes. On acount of the length of these processes, the number of muscles attached and the mobility of the articulations, torsion of the atlas and occiput on the axis from muscular contractions often occurs. These muscles contract from thermic influences. This form of stimulation most often affects the neck. Nature provides against this by giving man hair which, covering the neck, protects it against exposure. Fashion has decreed that the hair should be worn closely cropped and as a result one of nature's defences is weakened. In the male the throat is protected in a similar manner by hair on the face.

In man, contractures come in the neck from direct trauma, thermic stimuli, and toxemia, etc., by which the cells are over stimulated; and from lesions of the neck by which the nerve trunks are stimulated, the nerve cells irritated and the muscles put on a stretch on account of change in position of the origin or insertion. It seems that a muscle undergoes a change in structure as a result of prolonged stimulation of its nerve, which condition is readily recognised on palpation as muscular contracture.

When these muscles remain contractured for any great length of time the vertebrae are abnormally approximated, hence the intervertebral foramina are smaller, the circulation through the muscle impaired and, consequently, the blood supply to the cervical spinal cord, medulla and pons varolii interferred with. The nerve filaments passing through and in relation with, the contractured muscle, are also affected. On the other hand, lesions affecting the innervation of these muscles produce contracture, which in turn produces the above effects.

The structures affected by vertebral lesions in order of frequency are the ligaments, veins, arteries, nerves and muscles.

The veins in relation with the atlas are the vertebral and rami spinales which collect the blood from the upper cervical segments of the spinal cord and the spinal column. In lesions of the occipito-atlantal articulation there is pressure on these veins since they are in close relation with it. The result of a lesion would necessarily be a venous disturbance in the parts drained by the vessels that are compressed. This venous congestion affects nutrition of nerve cells located in the affected segments, hence an atlas lesion, by affecting drainage of the first and second cervical segments, disturbs the function of the nerves arising from them.

The vertebral arteries are affected by a lesion of the occipito-atlantal articulation. Pressure on these arteries is the most common effect. As a result the parts supplied by the artery are likely to be affected unless the anastomosis is complete, which is almost impossible on account of the branches being end arteries. The parts to suffer are the spinal cord and its coverings, medulla pons, cerebellum and quite a large part of the cerebrum, especially the centres for vision. Recalling the functions of these parts one can readily see an explanation for distrubances of the eye and other parts whose nerves have their cells of origin here. Vaso-motor nerves accompany and control the size of these arteries. The source of the nerve energy transmitted by these nerves is at a point below, perhaps in the upper thoracic segments of the spinal cord.

The nerves directly in relation with the atlas are the cerebro-spinal nerves and their branches and communications, coming from the first and second cervical segments – the sympathetic gangliated cord with some of its branches and communications – and the vertebral plexus. The anterior and posterior divisions and grey ramus with the vaso-motor nerves of the lateral spinal arteries carry impulses that pass through the intervertebral foramen between the occiput and atlas, while the gangliated cord with its ganglia and branches are in relation with the transverse processes.

In all lesions affecting the occipito-atlantal articulation the sub-occipital nerve is involved. This nerve supplies the rectus capiti, obliqui, complexus, genio-hyoid and infra-hyoid muscles. It supplies the mastoid process of the temporal bone, the occipito-atlantal articulation and in some cases sensation to the back part of the head. Some say that it helps to supply the meninges of the brain. It communicates directly with the 2nd cervical nerve, the 9th and 12th cranial, the superior cervical ganglion and the vertebral plexus around the vertebral artery.

I apologise for taking up so much of your time with this applied anatomy;

nevertheless, I think you will agree that Dr Clark makes the subject much more interesting than the average text book.

As to the actual mechanics of this articulation, writers such as J.M. Littlejohn, Webster, Hoover, Guy, Beckwith, Fryette and others, have made much contribution and all of these have acknowledged Fryette's *'Physiological Movements of the Spine'* as the basis for spinal mechanics, and the behaviour of these mechanics under stress. J.M. Littlejohn and Webster expressed their opinions further by utilising the three point support theory (the Tripod Principle) that each vertebrae from the 5th lumbo-sacral to the axis represents the support for the vertebrae above it, i.e. the three points of support are:

1. The nucleus pulposis between the bodies, together with the body of the vertebrae as the foundation support.
2. The two articulating facets as the accessory physical supports. The law of this principle of movement demands that "the weight must always be borne by one leg of the Tripod, because this is the only way in which to change the relative position between foundation and weight. If two legs of the Tripod were in contact with the foundation, relative movement on that foundation would be difficult except in connection with sidebending." The only possible alteration to this law is found in the occipito-atlantal articulation where the imposed weight (of the head) is borne by two foundation supports representing compression on the condyles of the atlas with the third leg represented by the ligamentum nuchae; this, in treatment terms, means that all stresses below the occipito-atlas-axis area must be removed if possible, to give the greatest degree of relaxation to the ligamentum nuchae and muscles originating from this point, e.g. the trapezius, for the maintenance of any correction of these articulations.

It is impossible to consider causes of C. lesions without considering the spine as a whole. Few people have spines that are in perfect balance, laterally or anterior-posteriorly. The head always tends to adjust itself to the line of gravity. Furthermore, it is a fact that all four movements general to the spinal column in flexion, extension, rotation and sidebending are distributed between the occipito-atlas-axis area as specific and characteristic main foundation movements, i.e. the characteristic movements between the occiput and the atlas are *Flexion* and *Extension* with minimum rotation and sidebending = maintenance of lesion = minimal movements.

The characteristic movement of the atlas is rotation with minimum flexion and extension and sideshifting, and the characteristic movement of the axis is sidebending with minimum rotation and flexion.

The distribution of the major movements of the spine among the three uppermost articulations must represent the answers to some of the difficulties that are experienced in the adjustment of the occipito-atlantal joint.

J.M. Littlejohn always insisted that flexibility must always be obtained from below up before attempting adjustment of this area.

Fryette simply states "The occipito-atlas-axis - axis-third have a very profound, subtle and, to me, still, a very mysterious relation." But, he goes on to describe the keypoint in adjustment of this articulation by saying, "Many years ago I leant from sheer accident and desperation that when this upper cervical group are in lesion, the key to the whole combination may be with the axis on the the third." He stressed this to me when I first met him 30 years ago, and I have yet to prove this statement wrong. Certainly equal attention should be paid to the cervical musculature, especially the larger muscles which affect chiefly the postural control of the neck as a whole from the shoulder to the occiput – muscles such as the trapezius, sterno-cleido-mastoid, longus colli, splenius capitis, the scaleni, etc.

These should be studied alongside the smaller muscles which control the individual upper cervical articulations. A lesion here (O-A) represents more strain through the effort of the central nervous system to balance and co-ordinate the contraction of muscles pulling on the vertebrae.

Just allow me to repeat "The head always tends to adjust itself to the line of gravity." This is accomplished by accommodation movements within the occipito-atlantal articulation via the condyles – outside of direct or indirect trauma (such as whiplash injuries) – the occipito-atlas lesion is secondary or compensatory to stresses below the axis, and should be examined in diagnosis with this in mind. It will save the osteopath much time and exasperation, and it will save the patient much mental and physical stress. I say this despite the paragraph in Dr Fryette's book on *'Principles of Osteopathic Technic'*, which is headed 'One's success in treatment is governed very largely by one's diagnosis'. I quote "It is very easy to locate a spinal segment that is in lesion, and to 'bust' into it with enthusiasm, and *hope* that part, at least, of what is done will be right." "Sad to say, by the grace of the *Divine Essence* which operates our bodies, this type of diagnosis and treatment sometimes does more good than harm. It seems to be so much easier for most of us to spare the brains and use the muscles."

I think the operative word here is *sometimes*, don't you?

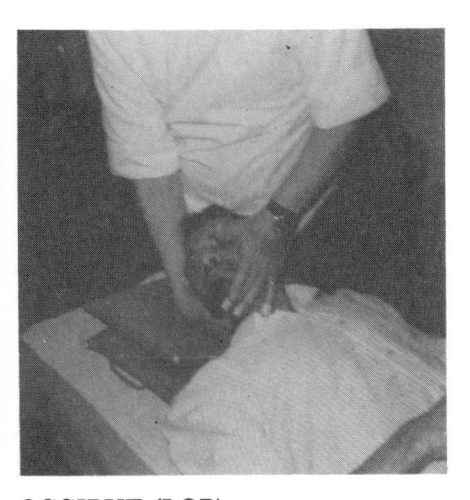

OCCIPUT (LOP)
Stabilised Atlas technique.
Thrust over the stabilised Atlas.

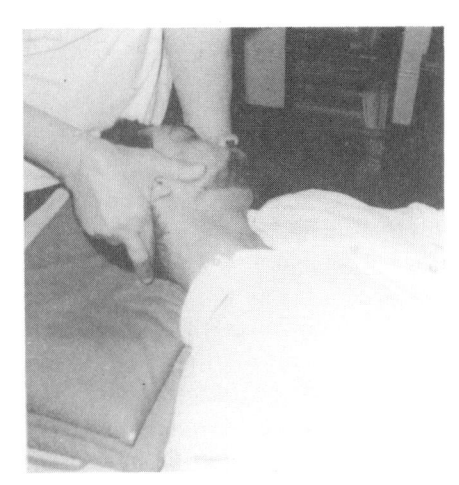

OCCIPUT (LOP)
Stabilised Atlas technique.
Showing crossed fingers to stabilise Atlas.

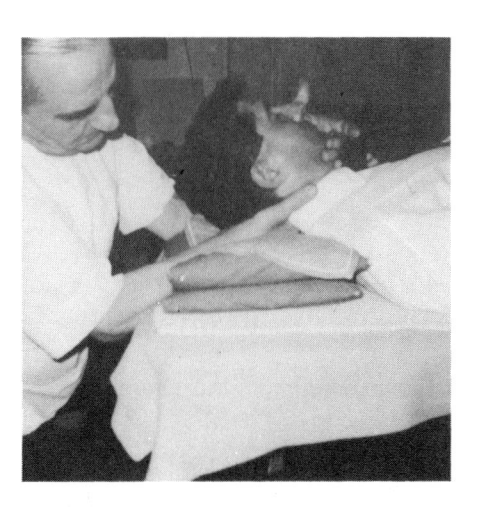

NECK TRACTION
Table fulcrum.

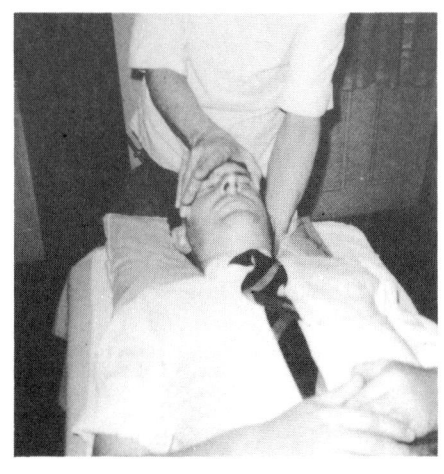

O / A ROCKING

THE ELBOW

The term 'tennis elbow' is on a par with all those other peculiar terms we hear, 'frozen shoulder', 'slipped disc', etc.

Diagnosis is or should be a process of elimination, which goes under the name, differential diagnosis, and if we spend a little more time on diagnosis, we would spend a sight less time working on the patient – we would not have to work on them for hours. We should be giving the right treatment based upon a correct diagnosis.

Pain in the elbow, forearm, wrist and hand can be due to many local and remote conditions, and demands as thorough an investigation as you would give to any other part of the body.

I would like to give you a few of the conditions which give rise to direct or indirect pain in this area.

(1) Carpal tunnel syndrome (often mistaken for a 'tennis elbow'), an affliction of the median nerve which arises from the 5th, 6th and sometimes 7th cervical nerves. This can give rise to pain in the tendons of the forearm and 'pins and needles', or paraesthesia, in the thumb.

(2) Capsulitis of the wrist – remember capsules have a reference of pain.

(3) Cervical lesion – the pain can be referred direct to below the elbow into the wrist and hand.

(4) Tendonitis of the supraspinatus – that can bypass the elbow and give pain down to the thumb.

(5) Tendonitis due to direct trauma.

(6) Tenosynovitis with or without stenosis – with stenosis the feel is of crackling all the way down the tendon, as you go on treating the case that crackling ceases and you know you have restored your tendon sheath.

(7) Capsulitis of the elbow – very seldom thought of, but the elbow has quite a large capsule.

(8) Bursitis, e.g. the bursa under the tendon of the biceps at its insertion into the radial head. This bursa is often in trouble and is also called a 'tennis elbow' by some.

(9) Tearing (pulling) strain of the biceps tendon, e.g. if you suddenly lift a heavy load.

(10 Fibrositis of the fascia that covers the whole of the lower third of the biceps tendon and over its insertion. That, following injury, can be very troublesome and has to be given some very deep soft tissue treatment.

In all cases a thorough examination of the area from the 4th cervical to the 4th dorsal is important.

Unlike the knee joint which has no reference of pain from itself the elbow has a great reference of pain down the arm.

The most common osteopathic lesions around the elbow are those associated with direct or indirect injury, involving the head of the radius, the ulna, and the distal end of the humerus, and includes the capsule as well.

The principle change that occurs is a proximo-distal movement between the radius and ulna, in which the radius moves upward along the long axis of the ulna. Upon first thought this seems to be impossible, because the rounded concave head of the radius is constantly applied to the lateral articular surface of the distal end of the humerus, which we call the capitulum. But it is not difficult to explain if you know your movements of the elbow. The olecranon in the olecranon fossa has a sideways movement in both directions. It is usually in lesion (7 times out of 10) in the adduction position, where the olecranon process is jammed into the medial side of the olecranon, and it stays there, and it has no lateral movement. Now when the elbow does that, it leaves the radial head with the capsular ligament away from the capitulum, and sooner or later, leaves a potential distance between the radial head and the capitulum. So, sooner or later you get the radius riding upwards and the capsular ligament becomes thickened. It also effects eventually, if you do not shift it, the carrying angle of the hand on the wrist so that it is not long before you get pain in the wrist – in fact the patient may come in for pain in the wrist. When the elbow is semi-flexed, the medio-lateral movement of the humeral joint, (that is the olecranon process within the olecranon fossa) is absent, flexion/extension is slightly limited and forceful extension or flexion is accompanied by pain.

This means that the lesion is a composite one consisting of adduction of the ulna upon the humerus, taking up all the free lateral movement between these bones and permitting a potential interval to occur between the proximal end of the radius and the capitulum of the humerus. The radius then moves upwards along the long axis of the ulna and remains fixed there by the same factors which maintain lesions in any other part of the body.

If this lesion is left unattended it is going to be accompanied by an anterior or posterior movement of the head of the radius; most commonly anteriorly, but this is not always as obvious as the less common posterior movement of the radial head.

This anterior/posterior movement is a factor which is most readily recognized when present, and is more often than not considered the most important diagnostic point, and accounts for the classification in commonse use, i.e. the anterior or posterior radius.

It is difficult to imagine that any of these lesions can exist if there is free and normal movement in the olecranon fossa of the olecranon process.

The lesion that our medical friends think of as 'tennis elbow' (and that is the only thing that they think about) is some injury by tear or strain or stress at the teno-periosteal junction on the lateral epicondyle of the humerus.

If you get a bad teno-periosteal junction, that has been neglected until you get tendosynovitis and vaginitis in your extensor muscles of your forearm, you probably start getting symptoms of a carpal tunnel syndrome and it is very difficult to diagnose and treat.

A differential diagnosis can be helped by asking the patient to point to the pain. If they point to the lateral epicondyle your prognosis is gradual recovery. But if they point to the radial head or below it ($1/4$ inch) you know you have a mechanical problem and your prognosis is better. Within that $1/4$ inch is the difference.

DO'S AND DON'TS IN TREATMENT

(1) Never cause pain – with possible exception of an acute meniscus it is bad osteopathy to cause pain during treatment. Speed, timing, etc. are used to avoid pain – you may cause shock or surprise but not pain.

(2) Never fight a lesioned articulation – if you do you will bruise deep tissues – you should go away from these apparently incorrectable lesions. Treat above and below and never go at it without preparation.

(3) Never adjust from a static position. If you grip it the patient will not relax. If you are static you will not get an adjustment, you will either damage yourself or the patient or both. You must adjust from a moving state.

(4) Never send a telegram to your patient – or even a postcard!

N.B. Fryette had a saying: "If a patient comes in and points with his finger 'there is the pain' – then this is a nerve pain. If he comes in and says, 'the pain is all over there' and he puts the whole of his hand over it – it is usually vasomotor in origin, (no matter what part of the body is concerned), and you have to get back to your sympathetics 2D - 2L."

TESTS FOR ELBOW MOVEMENT

In diagnostic movements of the elbow (like any other joint) the movements should be confined to the elbow and not involve the shoulder.

(1) Take the wrist and put it under your arm, hold the arm so the elbow can flex. You get behind the tip of the radius and then put the arm in

extension and flexion and see if they move forward and backward equally.

(2) Change the position of your finger on to the posterior head of the radius and just allow the elbow to drop into flexion.

(3) From there, still keeping your finger between the capitulum and the head of the radius just extend them and see if they both return equally and without trouble.

(4) Put your thumb over the head of radius anteriorly and your finger between the radius and capitulum, just apply downward pressure and let it relax. You will feel the head of the radius separating and going backward and forward on the capitulum. You note the difference, whether one is sluggish, posterior or anterior.

(5) Then with your fingers between the radial head and the capitulum, allow them to flex, which will allow them to open, and then extend them which will close them up. Note any oddities or differences between the two. If you have a posterior lesion it will not fully extend. If anterior, the head of the radius will "almost disappear".

(6) Test for movement of the olecranon process in the olecranon fossa.

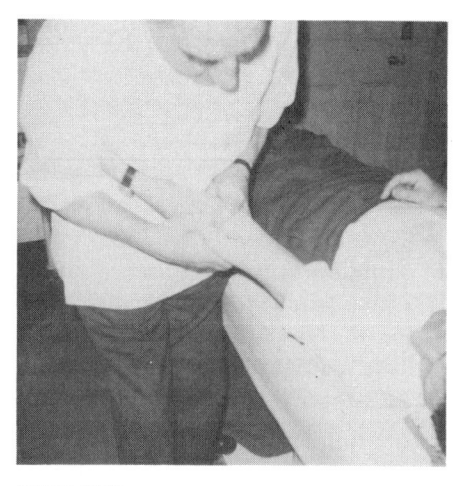

ELBOW
Circumduction, adduction.

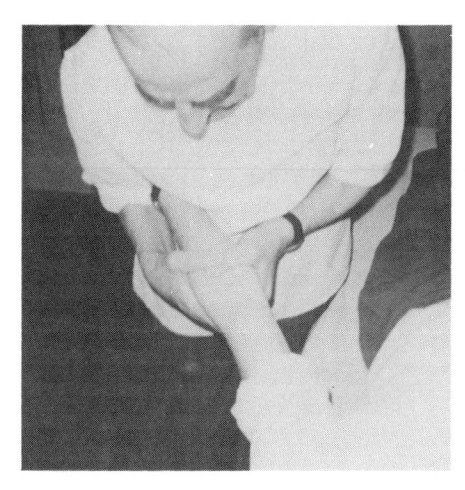

ELBOW
Circumduction, abduction.

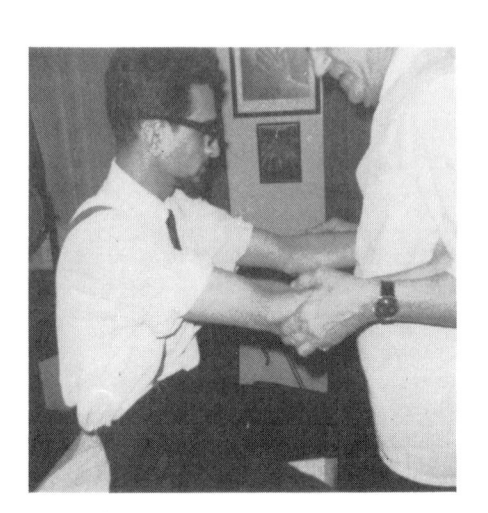

ELBOW
Comparing movement on both sides.

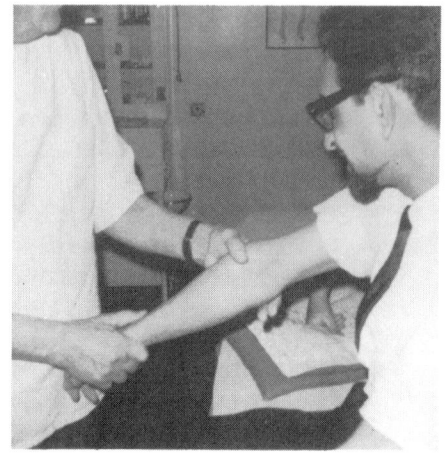

ELBOW
Correction grip.
N.B. *Ability to rotate radius (supination/pronation) and ability to abduct, adduct and extend from this grip.*

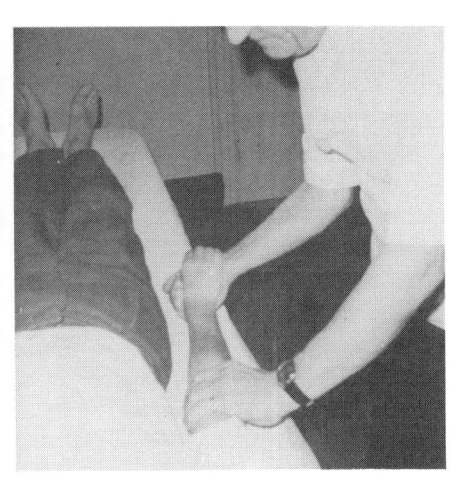

ELBOW
Supination and pronation.

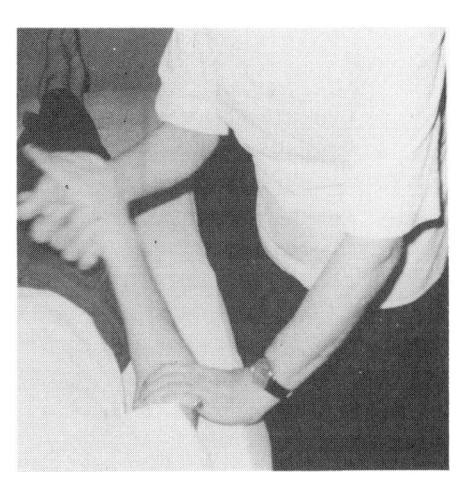

ELBOW
Supination and pronation.

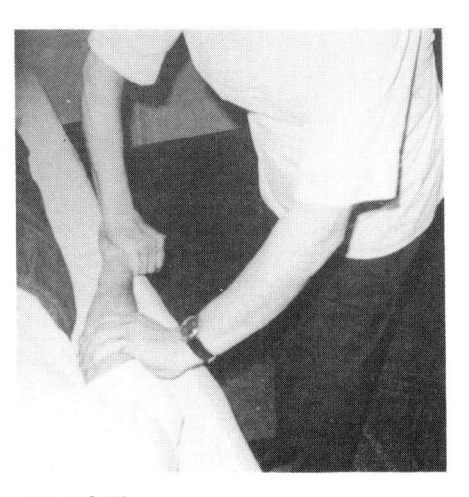

ELBOW
Supination and pronation.

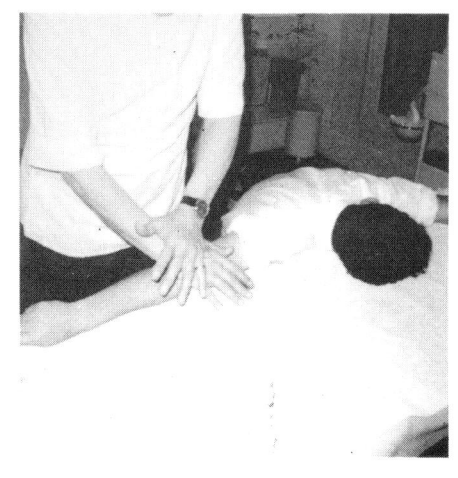

ELBOW
Prone technique for a olecranon lesion (double thrust).

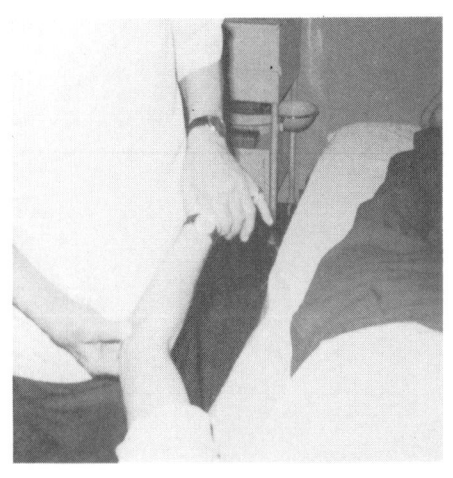

POSTERIOR RADIUS
Slap against thigh technique 1.

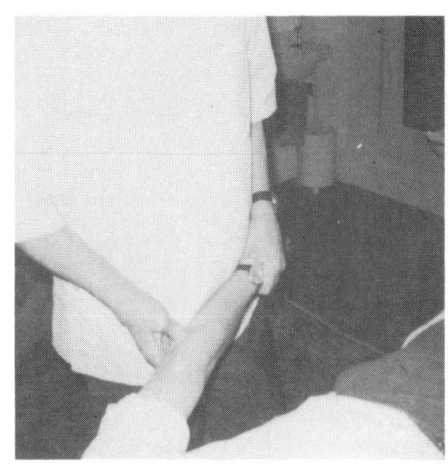

POSTERIOR RADIUS
Slap against thigh technique 2

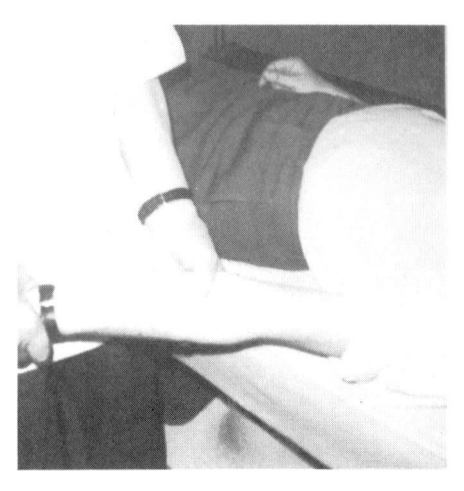

POSTERIOR RADIUS
Gapping and hyper extension with thrust over radial head.

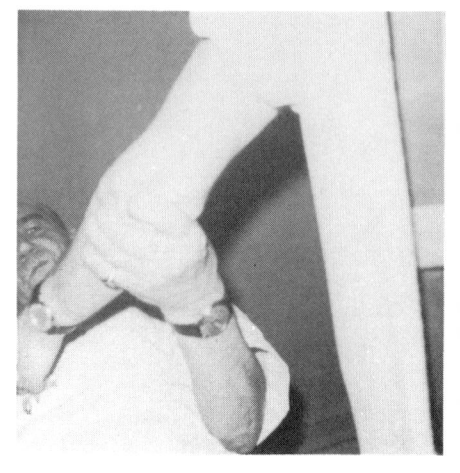

POSTERIOR RADIUS
Gapping and hyper extension (from below).

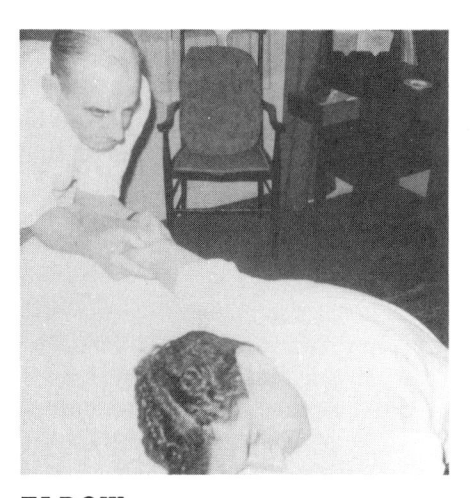

ELBOW
Prone technique.
Circumduction and down thrust.

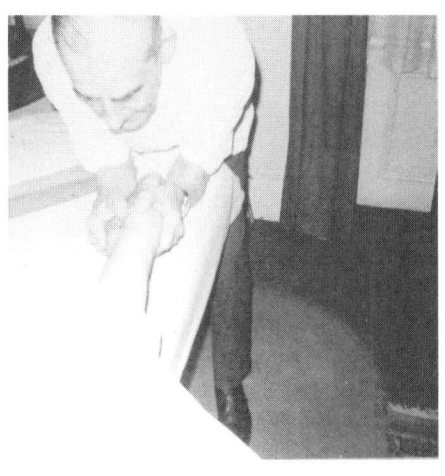

ELBOW
Circumduction and down thrust.

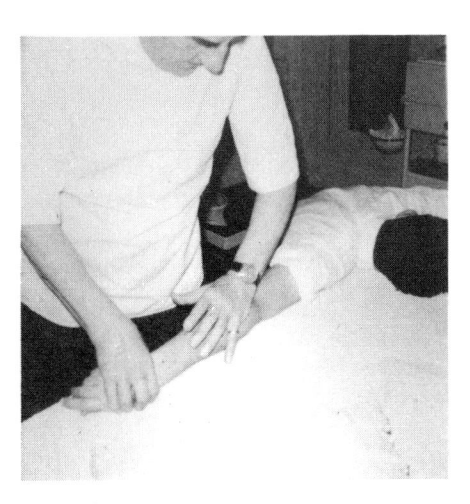

ELBOW
Prone technique.
Single thrust with supination.

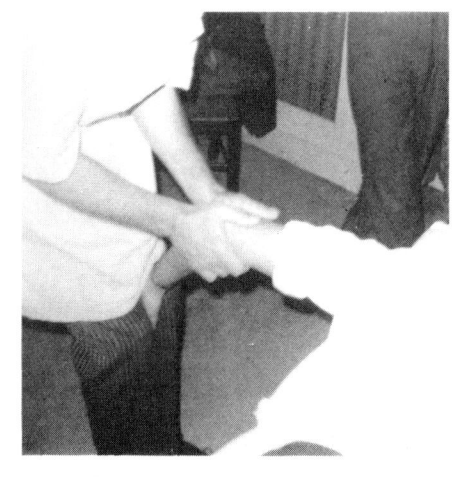

ELBOW
Knee hold technique. Elbow articulation. Circumduction and correction under traction.

THE SHOULDER
'FROZEN SHOULDER'

The reason why I have chosen this subject is to try to differentiate pain in the shoulder from the many conditions which are lumped together under the stupid term 'the frozen shoulder'. We are so used to hearing this, that we are in great danger of accepting this loose terminology as fact, as we accept the diagnosis of tennis elbow, slipped disc, or to our sorrow sometimes, sprained wrist.

The frozen shoulder is on the way out, except for one or two specific conditions, especially since hydrocortisone came in as a form of treatment applied in the acute or active stage. The causes of frozen shoulder have been discussed every five years over the last 60 years with a different cause each time, which was believed to be true at that time. I must speak to you about the biceps tendon, and bursitis of the sub-deltoid and subacromion bursa in relation to frozen shoulder, especially if calcification is present. In fact there is seldom a specific cause laid down by the patient, other than direct or indirect trauma, and these do not necessarily give rise to the real frozen shoulder.

It is necessary to divide the main causes of pain in the shoulder into four main categories. I except, fractures, dislocations, disease or congenital conditions.

(1) The first of these conditions represented as a frozen shoulder is the mono-articular rheumatoid type of capsulitis, which is usually arthritic with a toxic background.

(2) Traumatic capsulitis, is the second condition; it is a partial capsulitis with a possible tear in the capsule and adhesions giving rise to pain and limitation of movement.

(3) Referred conditions through to the dermatomes; i.e. osteopathic lesions; pressure on the nerve roots, inflammatory oedema around the articular facets, lesions in the discs or cartilages. Here we must remember that the deeper the structures involved the further will be the reference of pain to the dermatomes, (the 'constant length phenomena').

(4) Injury to muscle, tendon and local structures. Here the limitation of movement is voluntary by the patient because of actual localised pain in the contractile tissues and inert tissues. No direct pain is present except under muscle control and subsequent movement.

A small stimulus represents a small amount of pain. While all these conditions integrate to a certain extent and certain symptoms are common to all, it is up to us to isolate them and attempt to arrive at a differential diagnosis. This is absolutely essential if we are to be able to give specific and correct treatment, advice for the quick recovery of the patient and a controlled prognosis.

Now let us take the first of these:

(1) The Mono-articular Rheumatoid Capsulitis

This is of arthritic origin and a possible toxic focus of infection present somewhere in the body, which, of course, must be searched for and eliminated. It is associated, in many ways with an acute form of spondylosis in the spine and indeed in any other joint.

We find the gleno-humeral joint is relatively limited in local mobility and when pain is present, it is constant from any angle of movement, and from the very commencement of that movement. We can be sure we are dealing with a case of what we call a frozen shoulder, or what we call here a mono-articular rheumatoid capsulitis. The driving mechanism of the joint is interferred with, and pain and decrease of movement increases in proportion and keeps on to proportionate limitation in movement.

The history of onset in these cases is difficult to access. In fact the patient is not conscious of any known cause. He may say that weeks or months ago he felt something in the forearm or around the deltoid muscle insertion but it passed away. Nobody seems to know the real cause of this painful type of shoulder. It has been said to follow some operations, neck or coronary conditions, and upper rib conditions. The E.S.R. is usually slightly raised as indeed it should be with some infection present.

These are the cases, which, before the introduction of hydrocortisone were left to recover by what must surely facetiously be known as 'spontaneous recovery'. They were expected to be pain free and almost fully mobile within 16 months to 2 years. We, as osteopaths, and without hydrocortisone, are expected to do better than this, and indeed we do. But, I assure you, I have had shoulder cases which have not recovered within a reasonable time, and I think the answer lies in them being this particular type of painful shoulder. Perhaps one which we did not recognize from the beginning, and neither did anyone else, until the condition was established.

It is certainly insidious in its onset with perhaps the patient remembering a vague pain usually somewhere around the deltoid insertion which then went away. This is usually the beginning, when the stimulus of slight inflammation in some part of the shoulder, be it in capsule, muscle, ligament, tendon, leads to inflammatory oedema around the articulating facets. When this is present and when the stimulus is small, the reference of pain is small. As the stimulus and inflammation is increased we have the reference of pain going further down the arm until it reaches the dermatomes at the wrist or even the thumb. In other words, the greater the stimulus or the deeper the structures involved, the greater the pain length down the limb covering the dermatomes. This is

Cyriax's 'constant length phenomena' which we will refer to later.

This at least should give us a pointer as how to start the treatment of these cases. There has been worked out by Cyriax and others a pattern of diagnosis in these cases, called the capsular pattern. It is rather rough but accurate enough to give us a fairly constant pattern in a particular type of shoulder condition such as this.

Let us review what happens in cases such as this, where the patient is left to go on, untreated, to the 'spontaneous recovery'.

(a) First 4 months – the pain increases and movement decreases and there may be a spot of pain at the deltoid insertion.

(b) Second 4 months – there is still pain with the limitation of movement getting worse.

(c) Third 4 months – the pain settles down but the movement of the arm is very limited.

(d) Fourth 4 months – pain receding or almost gone but the range of movement still limited.

When cases come to you with this condition you must apply the capsule pattern test and marry the results with those of any other tests you do. This test reads:

(i) You hold the scapula and when abduction is tried it is found to be limited by 15° approximately.

(ii) From the side you try external rotation and find it is limited by 45° approximately.

(iii) When internal rotation is limited by putting the hand behind the back, it is limited by 5° approximately.

You can multiply these figures by two if abduction is doubled. You will notice that these figures are in multiples of three, i.e. 5, 15 and 45.

When you have this pattern it is an odds on chance that you will have referred pain down the whole length of the arm; a condition Cyriax called the constant length phenomena. This means that all the dermatomes below the shoulder are involved, and this means that you have constant pain below the elbow and into the wrist and hand. This in turn means there is still active inflammation in the capsule and three conditions exist which prohibit forced manipulation of the shoulder.

(i) When pain is felt below the elbow.

(ii) When pain is felt at rest.

(iii) When the patient cannot lie on the affected side.

This is the time when you should use hot and cold packs to the shoulder, pay more attention to the soft tissues in the neck and upper dorsal area, and apply very gently gapping traction to the gleno-humeral joint. This is als the time when hydrocortisone helps most, that is, during the active inflammatory condition.

When this constant length phenomena begins to recede you find that:
(a) There is no pain below the elbow
(b) There is no pain when at rest.
(c) There is no pain when the patient lies on the affected side.

It is then that full manipulative procedures are indicated, locally to the shoulder joint as such, and to the deep tissues and underlying lesions in the cervical area. By this time the patient himself is moving his shoulder freely and with your help will be very soon completely normal.

By the way, it is said that this condition never recurs in the same shoulder; that I wouldn't know, but this is your real "frozen shoulder".

(2) <u>Traumatic Capsulitis</u>

This is due to severe injury inflicted on the shoulder such as a sudden jerk on a bus especially if 'strap hanging', a sudden blow over the acromio-clavicular area from above, certain strain or stress applied to any or more of the muscles involved in the rotor cuff group or any of the external rotator group arriving from the spine to the shoulder. Even the latissimus dorsi can be involved here as a cause of pain in the shoulder.

If the trauma is severe it can even result in a tear in the capsule with adhesion formation not only in the capsule but also in the ligaments, tendons and bursae. Pain here is not necessarily due to capsulitis, but by the limitation of movement caused by injury to any of the above mentioned structures. Some disuse – atrophy may be obvious at this stage especially in the deltoid group.

In fact, this condition can reproduce most of the symptoms associated with the previous syndrome. If left untreated the pain may eventually go but the limitation of movement is worse owing to excessive muscular contraction and full recovery of normal movement is doubtful.

If necessary, tests must be carried out on each individual muscle for interference with function and conduction. Treatment here takes the form of local manipulation direct to the shoulder and to any individual muscle that you find involved, plus ancillary treatment by exercises such as weight swinging, wall crawling or towel pulling, or anything else you use yourself such as active, passive, or resistant isometric exercises or even a sling in certain conditions which will be mentioned later.

(3) <u>Osteopathic Lesions referred through to the dermatomes</u>

These can give rise to pressure on the dural investment covering the nerve roots or inflammatory oedema around the articular facets, ligaments, cartilages or discs. Here again, one must remember the deeper the structures involved the further is the reference of pain to the dermatomes. This points to the particular segment of the cervical-dorsal area which is the cause of the trouble. This condition is closely allied to No. 4.

(4) Injury to muscles, tendons, ligaments and surrounding structures

The limitation to movement here is voluntary on the patient's part because of localised pain in the contractile or inert structures. No direct pain is present except under muscle control and subsequent movement. The stimulus may be small and indicate that only one muscle or ligament is involved. Therefore, the reference of pain will be small and refer only to these structures and the treatment here must be obvious.

Examination of these cases can only be accepted as part of a differential diagnosis — we must find the underlying reason.

There are certain acute conditions allied to the shoulder that stand out conspicuously and are better dealt with by some form of specific treatment that is not necessarily adjustive as we understand the word. I refer, of course to a severe brachial neuritis, and to the inflamed condition and swelling of the sub-acromion and sub-deltoid bursa. You have all had cases of these conditions, and no doubt, have your own method of dealing with them.

But I would like to say that I have treated cases of brachial neuritis, severe and acute, by strong traction, in flexion on the McMurray table, by manipulation under anaesthesia and by all known osteopathic adjustive procedures to the lower cervical, and 1 and 2 dorsal vertebrae including the 1st and 2nd ribs, with a view to relieving not only nerve root and nerve trunk pressure, but also to try to normalise the scalenus anterior syndrome. which is in part responsible for this painful condition. I have had a very great percentage of good and permanent results by these various methods especially following specific adjustment of 2 and 4 dorsal vertebrae and accompanying ribs. But it is not always possible to use these methods because of:

(a) Age group — 40-70 years
(b) Constitutional condition
(c) Time limit
(d) Excessive size and obesity
(e) Chronic fibrositis condition in the deeper structure

Now over recent years, while attempting normalisation of the structures involved, I place my patient in a cuff and elbow sling, and in most cases guarantee complete relief from pain in 6 weeks even without osteopathic treament.

In acute cases of bursitis of the sub-acromion and sub-deltoid bursa with or without calcification, I also place the patient in a cuff and elbow sling and the patient is usually pain free within 10 days.

In both of these cases the patient is instructed to rotate the arm internally and externally while in the sling, which makes sure abduction of the arm is free when the sling is removed. Do please try these treatments before trying traction, manipulation or ruthless correction of the neck. Certainly in both cases it pays to examine the neck and give treatment to lesions as found, as long as the lesions are connected to the condition found.

Sometimes this sling idea when presented to the patient is not received with pleasure, but I can assure you, it works, and the patient will indeed be grateful afterwards.

SUMMARY

In the shoulder, as in any other joint, nothing is lost by a little patience in differential diagnosis. We must remember that local trouble in a muscle as such does not refer pain. Whereas trouble in tendons, ligaments or capsules do have a reference of pain to these dermatomes. Any tenoperiosteal junction has a great reference of pain, e.g. at the elbow joint.

We must check:

(1) Each muscle, separately if necessary, by passive, active and resisted movements
(2) The acromioclavaicular articulation
(3) The thoracic outlet, especially if the 1st rib is in lesion and the nerve trunk is involved
(4) Thoroughly for trouble anywhere between 4C and 4D
(5) For conduction loss and relate this amount of loss to the extent of pain and weakness found
(6) For weakness
(7) Wasting
(8) Alteration in sensation, e.g. 'pins and needles'
(9) Alteration in temperature (numbness or burning feeling)
(10) Anesthesia
(11) Paresthesia

If by our examination we find two or more spinal segments involved, particularly in reference to C6, 7 8, and T1 and 2 nerve roots, we should think very seriously of a differential diagnosis, between a root palsy, neuroma, posterior displaced disc and even a spinal tumour, especially if the nerve root damage refers pain to both arms.

FINDINGS WHEN TESTING AGAINST ISOMETRIC RESISTANCE
(1) Strong and painless – *nothing wrong*

(2) Strong and painful – *muscle lesion either in tendon, muscle-tendon junction or teno-periosteal junction*

(3) Weak and painful – *partial rupture or growth lesion in the muscle or bone*

(4) Weak and painless – *neurological condition; complete rupture of muscle or root palsy*

(5) All resisted movements weak in everything (even if painful or painless) – *may be psychological or again a growth bone lesion, (osteomyelitis or sarcoma)*

N.B .There are two principle sites for sarcoma – lower end of the humerus and lower end of the femur. Any growth lesion of a bone will give pain on movement due to the pull on the bone.

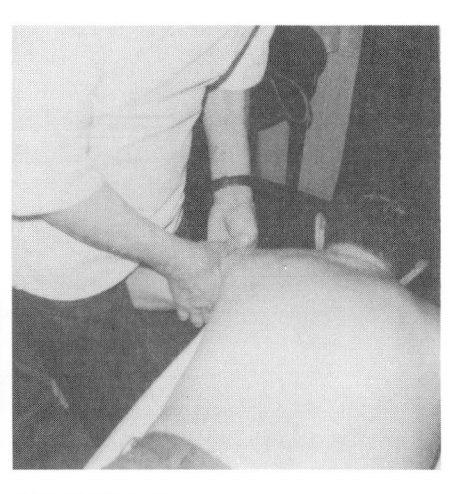

SHOULDER
Knee grip traction with mobilisation of humeral head.

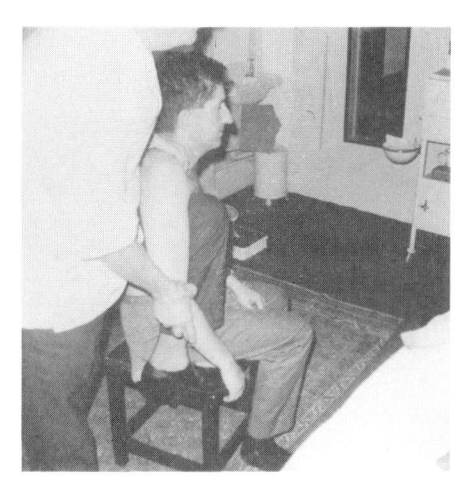

SHOULDER
Traction and gapping over knee.

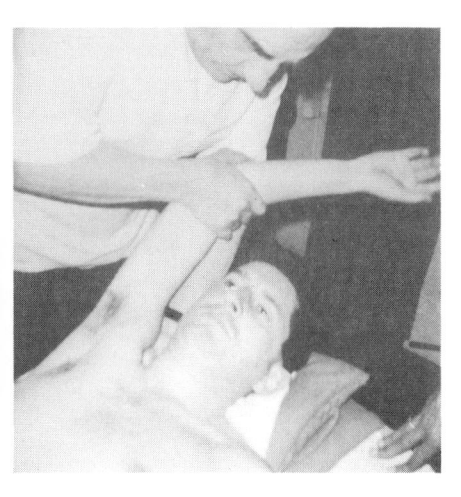

SHOULDER
Capsulitis

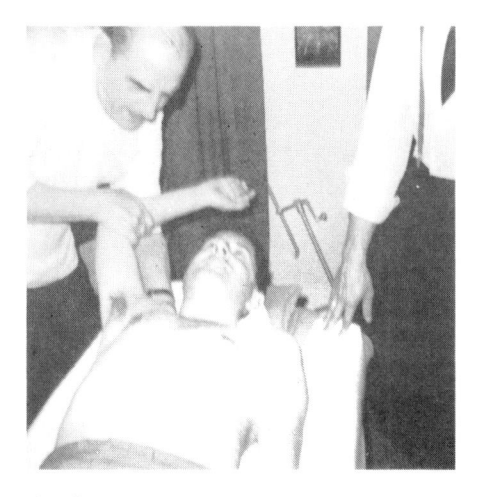

SHOULDER
Capsulitis

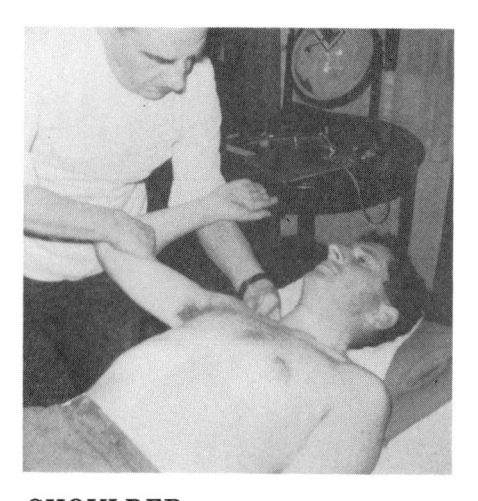

SHOULDER
Capsulitis

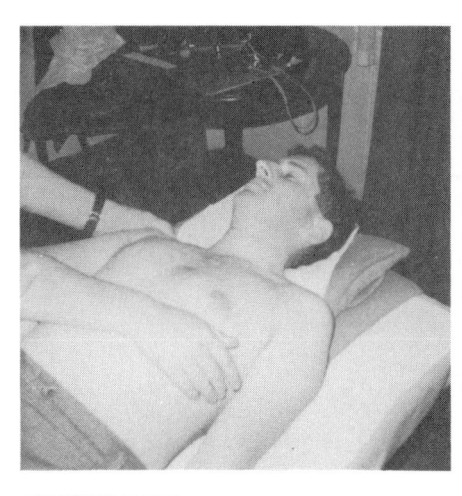

SHOULDER
Capsulitis

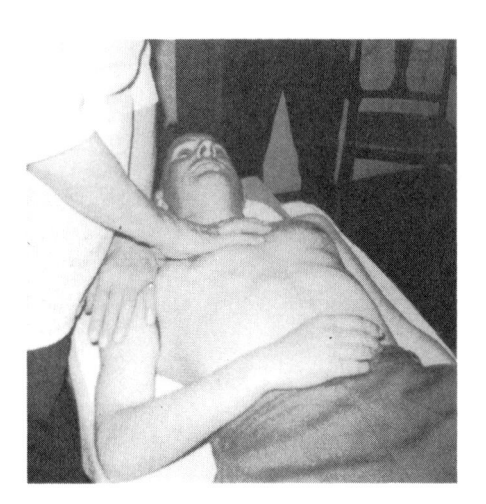

SHOULDER
Capsulitis
Supine cross hands thrust.

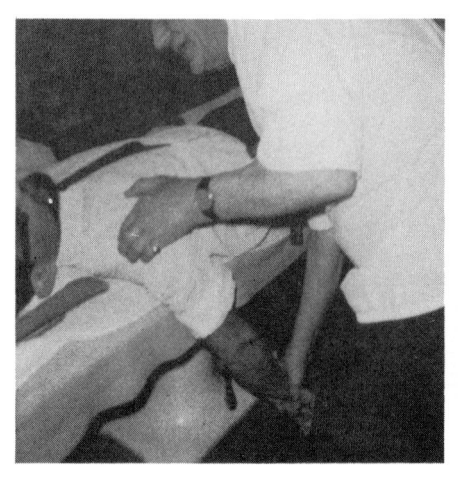

SHOULDER
Capsulitis
Supine technique

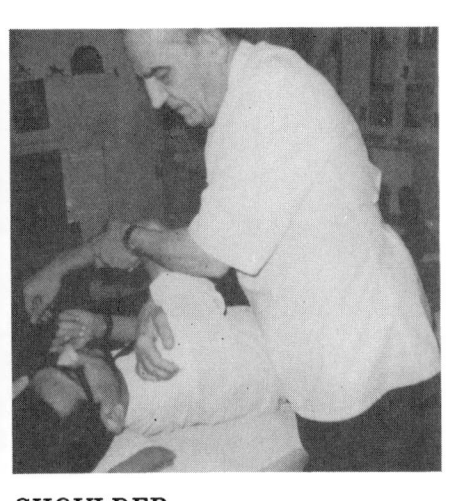

SHOULDER
Capsulitis
Supine technique

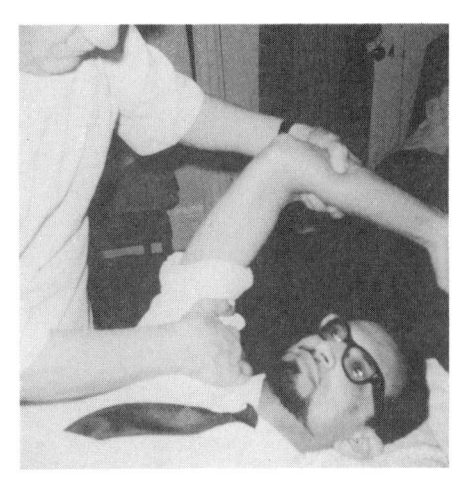

SHOULDER
Capsulitis
Supine technique

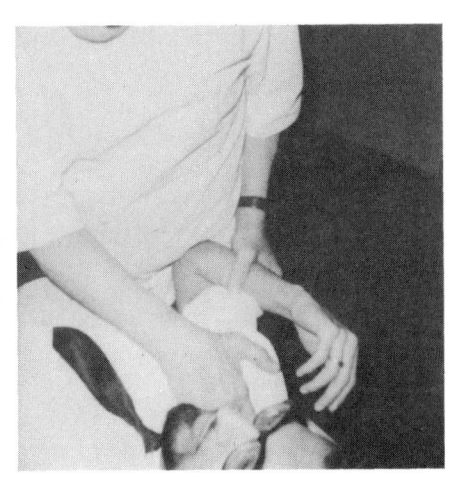

SHOULDER
Capsulitis
Supine technique

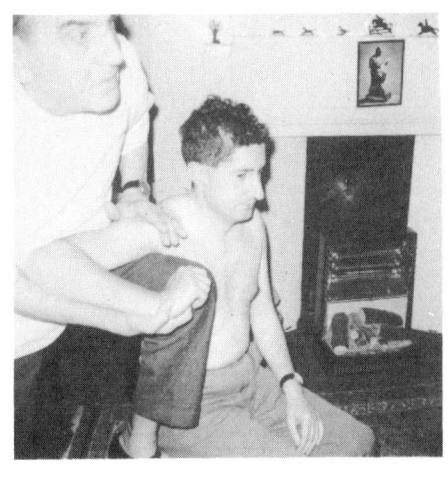

SHOULDER
Lateral elevation
Thrust over knee.

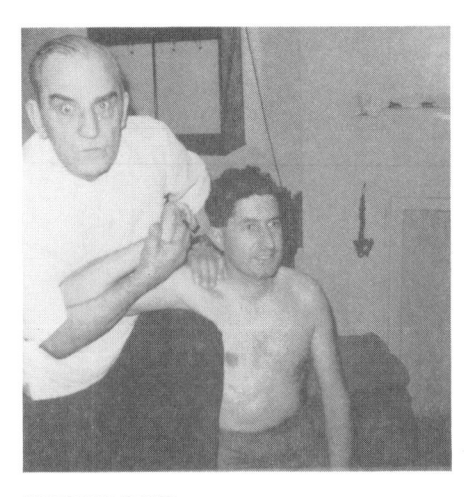

SHOULDER
Rotational thrust over knee.

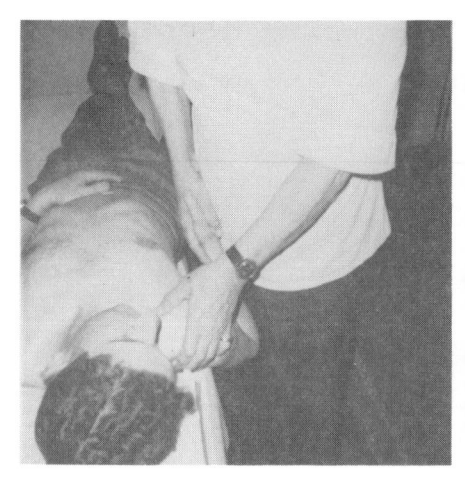

FROZEN SHOULDER
Manipulation under anaesthetic.
1

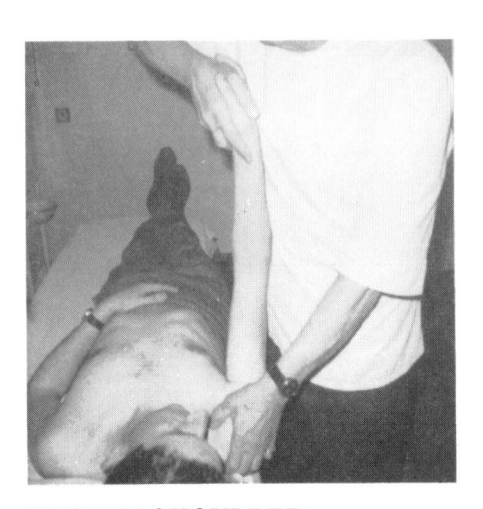

FROZEN SHOULDER
Manipulation under anaesthetic.
2

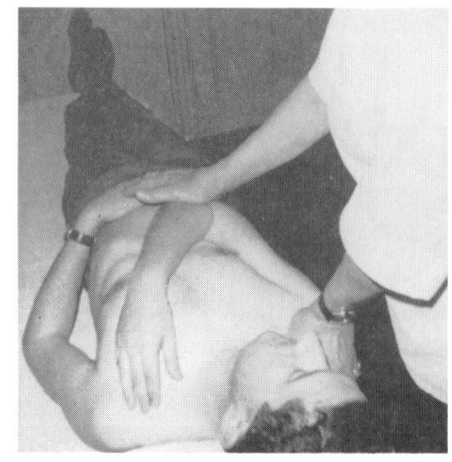

FROZEN SHOULDER
Manipulation under anaesthetic.
3

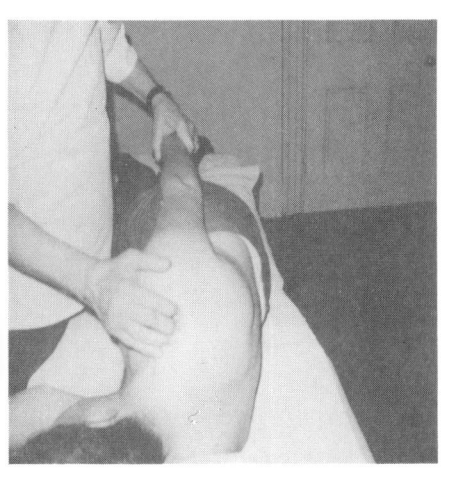

FROZEN SHOULDER
Manipulation under anaesthetic.
4

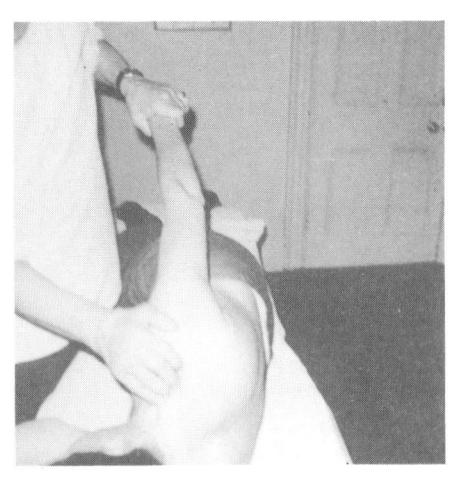

FROZEN SHOULDER
Manipulation under anaesthetic.
5

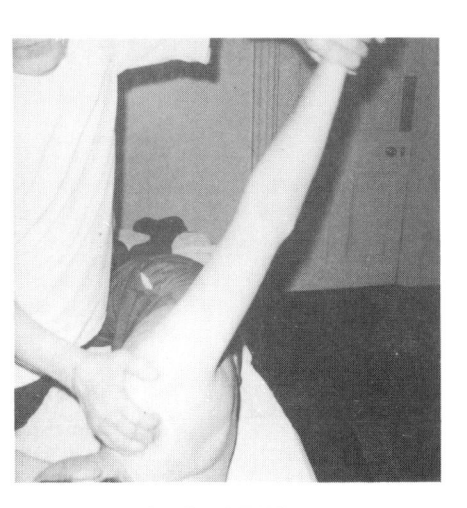

FROZEN SHOULDER
Manipulation under anaesthetic.
6

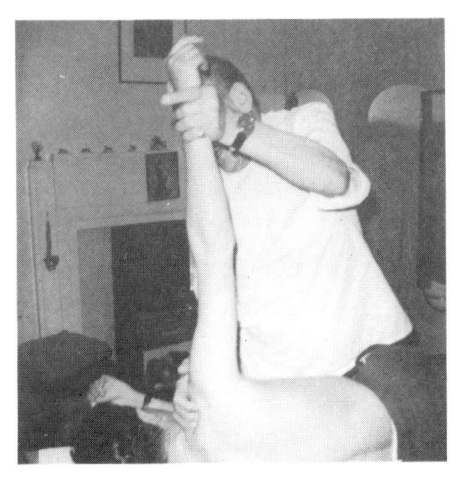

FROZEN SHOULDER
Manipulation under anaesthetic.
7

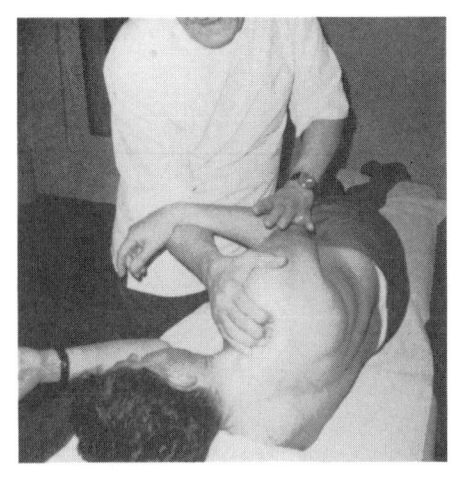

FROZEN SHOULDER
Manipulation under anaesthetic.
8

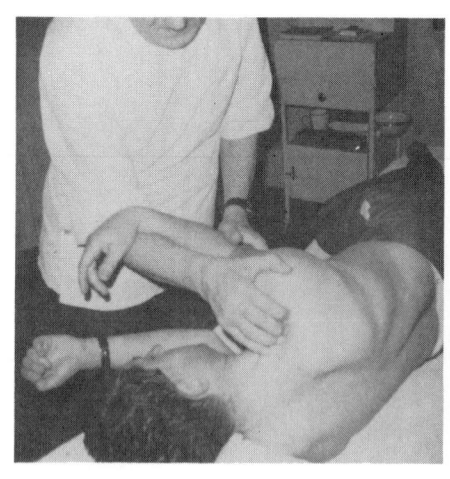

FROZEN SHOULDER
Manipulation under anaesthetic.
9

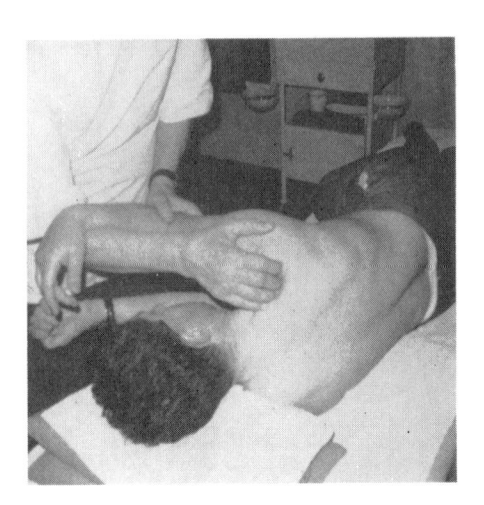

FROZEN SHOULDER
Manipulation under anaesthetic.
10

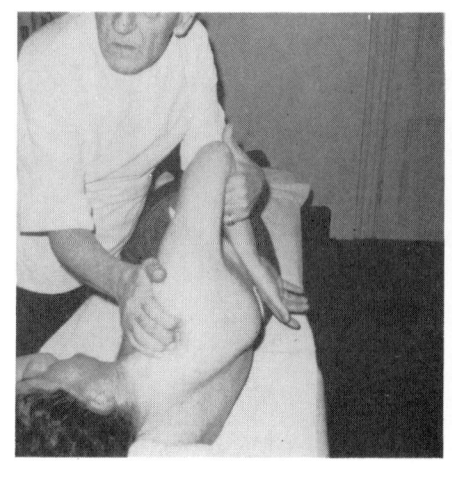

FROZEN SHOULDER
Manipulation under anaesthetic.
11

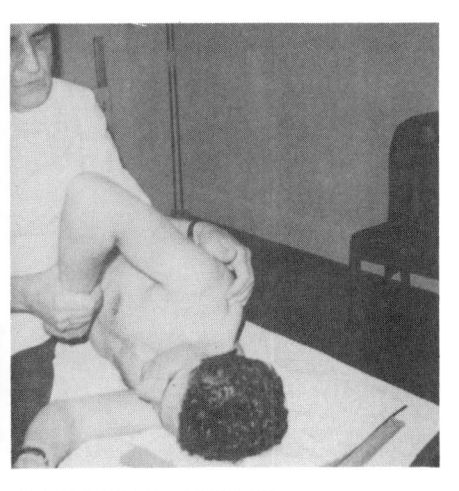

FROZEN SHOULDER
Manipulation under anaesthetic.
12

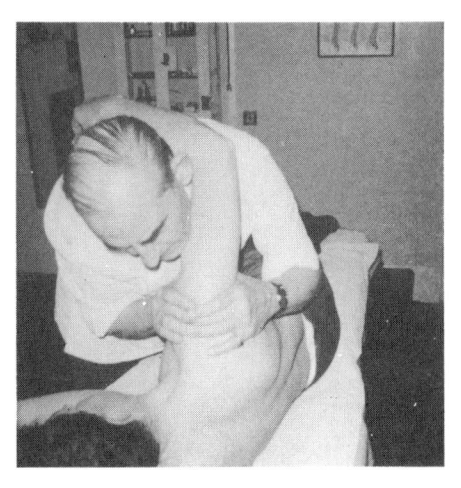

FROZEN SHOULDER
Manipulation under anaesthetic.
13

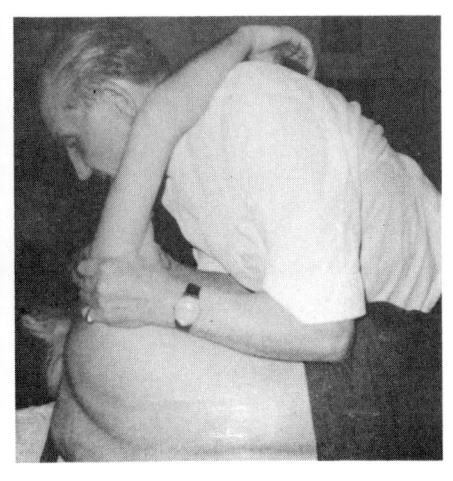

FROZEN SHOULDER
Manipulation under anaesthetic.
14

THE KNEE

Anatomically the stability of the knee is not due really to the apposition of the articular surfaces between the condyles of the femur and the tibia. It is not even held together with any strength at all by the capsular ligament and its extraneous ligaments, the collateral ligaments and the cruciates. It is held more or less together by the muscles that traverse the knee joint. These become tendons almost, like the biceps-femoris tendon inserted into the tibia and fibula. Out of about 16 muscles in the leg no fewer than 12 overlap the knee joint.

Of the anterior thigh muscles vastus medialis is the most important muscle as far as the knee is concerned. The quadriceps femoris is encapsulated over the patella, leading to the patella tendon which inserts into the tibial tubercle so that it is overlapping the whole line of the joint. You have posteriorly the powerful biceps femoris which inserts into the head of the fibula and some fibres cover the bursa of the popliteus muscle. This is important because you may have what appears to be a fibula lesion but by correcting the fibula you may be increasing injury to the popliteal bursa. It's a very powerful tendon and not only is it an extensor of the thigh it is an external rotator of the lower leg. Problems with this muscle tend to pull the fibula head posteriorly and superiorly as well as putting a drag on the popliteus. You also have the semi-membranosis which together with the bicipital tendon is a posterior flexor of the knee. The other muscles that traverse the knee joint are the origins of the gastrocnemeus which as you know joins up with the soleus muscle and then forms the common tendon of the Achilles tendon. The other muscle which is more or less often missed is the plantaris. This muscle has probably the longest tendon in the body, the actual muscle itself is possibly only $1/6$ th the length of its tendon which arises from the lateral posterior condyle of the femur and goes right down the side of the leg as a tendon to join in and support the Achilles tendon. The popliteal muscle arises from the same lateral posterior condyle of the femur and inserts into the fascia surrounding the tibia. There are 7 muscles covering the anterior medial aspect and 6 covering the posterior lateral aspect of the knee. These are the muscles that stabilise the knee joint.

I sat down the other day while thinking about this lecture and without looking through the text books, I came up with over 40 different causes of pain in the knee. There can be pain in the knee from any lesion of the pelvis but I won't deal with this today.

The knee joint is usually only associated with one lesion in the medical books; the displaced semi-lunar meniscus. Even so, if you read about the reduction of these cartilages, they are so contradictory! Some of these methods! A man with an acute cartilage would hit you before he would let you use them!

It requires confidence in your technique to reduce an acute cartilage. When a man comes in with a bent knee, on tip-toe, or on crutches with his foot off the floor, this is a difficult case. It depends on how well you know your technique and how willing you are to go through with it. I can teach you technique to correct any cartilage, but the acute episode is a thing you must look out for and be careful with.

As far as I'm concerned the knee is the most beautiful and fascinating joint in the body because it does such a lot of work. It has to compensate for any irregularities between the foot and the hip. Although anatomically the knee does not appear to be a stable joint, physiologically it is.

You must remember that the quadriceps group, through disuse atrophy can waste in circumference 1 inch in 24 hours. If you measure 6 inches above the patella, in a case where the patient has been hobbling around with pain in the knee joint, you will find about an inch difference in circumference between the two legs. If it's in the quadriceps generally, with isometric exercises you can bring that muscle back in a month with extensive treatment. If that case isn't taken care of in the first 3 days it can take up to 3 months to restore vastus medialis fully. Remember that the quadriceps cover the patella. Any damage to these muscles will result in minute haemorrhages in the area. Care must be taken to deal with these otherwise the patient will continue to complain of pain on weight bearing or flexion of the knee. Remember that vastus medialis takes care of the last 5-7% of extension in the knee. It doesn't come into use until then, so that when you test the knee joint, you must test it from every angle, test it from right angles to full extension, then take it down to nearly extension and resist the movement to full extension and if it hurts you know you have got a vastus medialis problem.

To understand the knee you must know your cartilages, not only their attachments but the anatomy of the cartilages on the tibial head. The movement of the knee joint is guided by the femur and controlled by the cartilages on the tibia. Don't bother to look them up in the ordinary anatomy books because they will say they are immovable. Well, they are not! Flexion and extension of the knee joint is governed by the femur, but torsion of the knee joint is governed by the movement of the cartilages on the tibial head. They have a certain amount of gliding motion on the tibial head itself, and this is responsible for one of the most common osteopathic lesions of the knee joint which is a lateral slip. This is a medial slip of the femur on the tibia but it is treated as a lateral slip of the tibia on the femur. You get rotation of the lower leg accompanying this which puts torsion on the cartilages, by the powerful pull on the biceps femoris. You must remember that the medial cartilage is by far the most important because not only does its collateral ligament arise from the medial portion of the condyle of the femur and is inserted into the medial portion of the tibia, but it is also attached to the synovial membrane. This is very important because any direct injuries of the medial aspect of the knee in a valgus direction can not only give rise to a displaced cartilage and a great deal of pain in the collateral ligament but it can also give rise to blood seeping into the joint.

Remember that the lateral cartilage is free to move much more extensively than the medial cartilage. It has been a long time since I have seen any severe strain of the lateral cartilage or collateral ligament. However it is in the lateral cartilage that you often find cases of cyst in the knee.

I hope you don't see many of these but if you do send them for surgery to be removed. Cysts on the medial side of the knee are very rare.

Always remember that the cartilages must be free to glide on the tibial head and that the movement of these cartilages is controlled by the condyles of the femur. What this means is, if there is any malposition of the femur on the tibia, any decrease of the range of cartilaganeous movement will predispose to an acute condition. If you get a sudden shearing, as you do occasionally in sportsmen etc., then a relatively minor degree of movement will produce a displaced cartilage.

If you don't restore the movement of the cartilages on the head of the tibia the knee is open to all sorts of trouble. This is a vital principle of treatment. You must realise that the cartilages are not static they are open to movement. The movement of the cartilages below the femur is that of torsion. The reason the medial cartilage is more often damaged is because of its attachments to the medial collateral ligaments and from the medial collateral ligament into the synovial membrane.

To try to reduce a lateral cartilage you must approach it a little differently from a medial cartilage because the lateral cartilage, through its two attachments posteriorly and anteriorly has more freedom of movement and it moves more frequently in a lateral direction when stress is put upon it. When you get a lateral cartilage come in you won't necessarily get pain over the cartilage. To reduce it you will have to get behind the lateral collateral ligament.

When examining the knee you must remember the posterior pad of fat behind the patella. Any blow on the patella tendon may cause haemorrage in the fat pad and lead to a haematoma and then you have got a "mystery knee". It apparently has full movement but pain is still felt when it is stressed.

You must also remember the bursae of the knee joint. You will have all had cases where there is swelling in the popliteal space. There is still some argument whether bursae communicate with each other but I believe that the popliteal bursae have means of communication.

In children you must be especially careful in examining the patella and patella tendon because of osteochondritis, osteomalacia etc. You must always ensure that the patella is completely mobile before attempting any adjustment of the knee joint.

In all cases watch out for the tibio-femoral misalignment – this is the osteopathic lesion of the knee. This is what we have contributed to the diagnosis of knee conditions and it is one of the most important and most often missed. It takes approximately two seconds to reduce! Next look at the proximal tibio-fibular articulation. Remember that any lesion of the fibula head must affect the fibulo-talus joint. Therefore if the head is posterior/superior it is anterior/superior at the fibio-talus joint. You will find the talus is jammed. Plantar flexion of the foot will be restricted.

In all knee problems do remember to examine the good knee. The patient may wonder what you are doing, but you should make sure that you put the normal knee through its range of movements first. Some people have a normal hyperextension etc., others don't. It is important that you know the patient's normal range of movement, especially flexion because you will often need to use forced flexion in your techniques.

You must be extremely careful in handling the acute knee, the patient must have confidence in you. A good approach is to fix the lower leg between your knees with the patient sitting on the table. This leaves your hands free for the examination but more importantly the patient knows that his leg is not going to be dropped. The one thing a patient is afraid of is the knee being allowed to drop as he knows it would be very painful. This does not apply so much to a patient with a chronic cartilage problem.

When putting a knee through its range of movement the first thing to do is to try flexion and extension; then initiate rotation and sidebending. For rotation hold the leg just below the right angle and rotate internally and externally. Make sure your fingers are on the joint line. If a lateral slip lesion is present external rotation will be full, but internal rotation will be only 50%. Couple this with the valgus and varus tests. These will correspond with the rotation tests if there is a lateral slip of the tibia on the femur. If you rotate medially and you get pain externally, the lateral coronary ligament is involved. If you rotate laterally and you get pain medially it is the medial cartilage involved. For the record, I can't remember when I last saw a lateral coronary strain, but I can remember a lot of medial coronary strains. Next test the cruciate ligaments. The anterior cruciate permits the joint to glide forward, the posterior, to glide back. If either of these have been strained and lengthened it makes for a very unstable knee joint. This often requires surgery.

Let me just mention a case I had recently. A man of 40 was sent to me by an osteopath from Manchester. He had great pain in the lateral aspect of the knee, with what appeared to be a cyst on extension. There was general swelling. It had me puzzled a bit, but I put him through the usual movements which he had no trouble with, but when I came to the cruciate ligaments they never budged a fraction of an inch. This was the only case I have ever seen of a locked cruciate ligament. When I got hold of the biceps femoris it was hard and tense. As I moved up the muscle he yelped. When we went into the history, he said that he had been trying to lift the bumper of his car off another car when he felt something give way on the outside of the knee joint. I decided that he had torn some of the fibres of the biceps femoris and the ilio-tibial fascia. I decided to stretch the cruciate ligaments and I did both, anteriorly and posteriorly. Then I went to work on the ilio-tibial band and the bicipital tendon. There was no extension of the knee and the leg was rotated outwards but once I stretched the tendons and cruciates, gradually full movement returned. Now, I almost sent that man for surgery as I had never seen anything like it before. If it wasn't for the fact that I always do a full examination of the joint and compare it with the good joint, I would not have been able to work out what was wrong.

Remember that with an acute cartilage the patient will not let you bend the knee while the quadriceps are on stretch, so the only way you can get flexion of the knee is by bringing the femur up to the chest. You can gradually increase it until you get full flexion, then by turning the knee in with a sudden full extension, the cartilage can be reduced. Hold the knee down and then test hyper-extension. If there is no pain the technique has been successful.

You should never hyper-flex the knee where there is fluid in the joint. Remember, if you get a swollen knee joint, the history is very important. If the swelling came up immediately it is most likely blood in the joint; if it took a few hours to come up it is synovial fluid. Blood in the joint should be drained off as soon as possible.

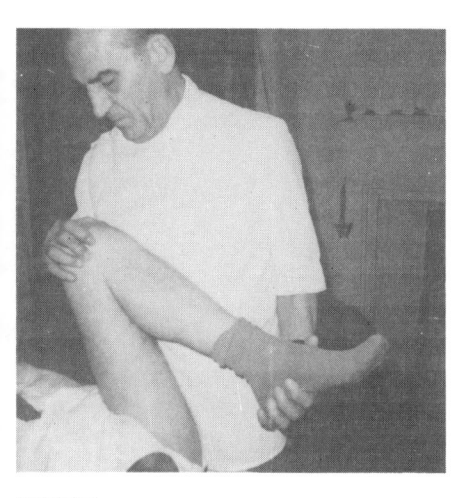

KNEE
Testing rotation of tibia on femur.

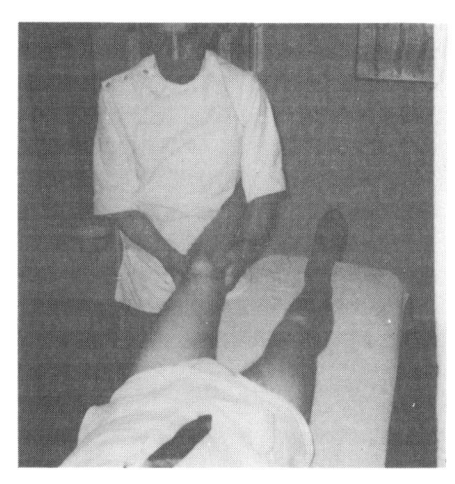

KNEE
Testing abduction and adduction.

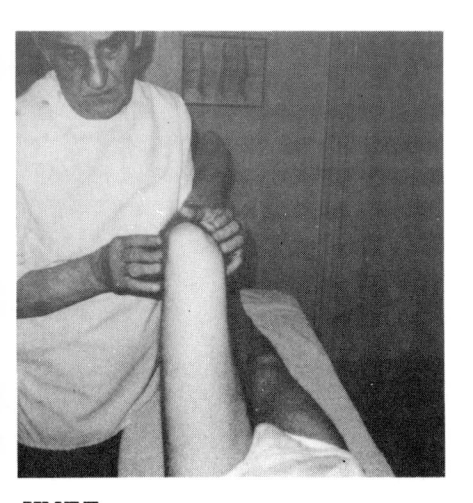

KNEE
Articulation and flexing before correcting medial cartilage.

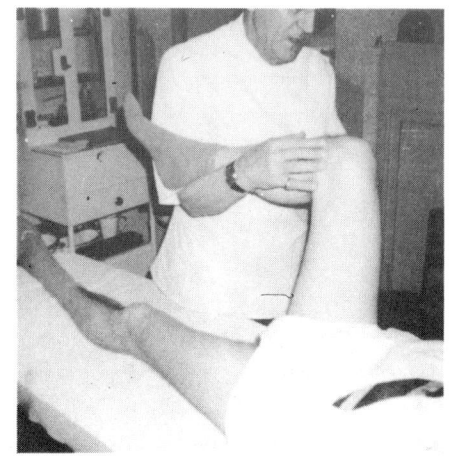

KNEE
Articulation (in flexion).

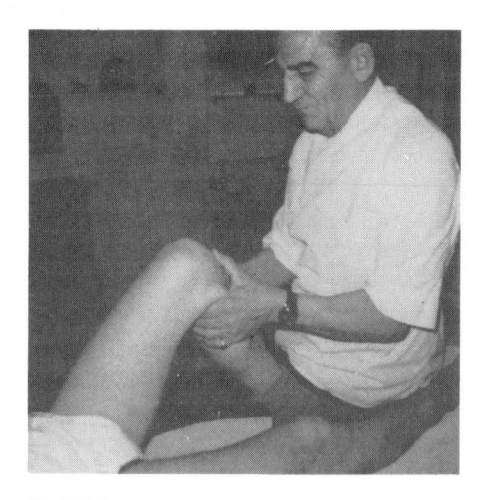

KNEE
Testing cruciates.

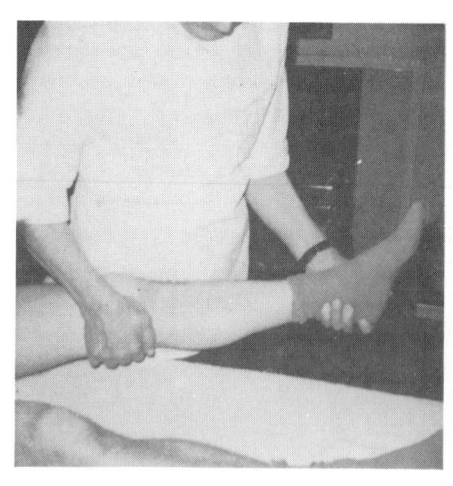

KNEE
*Lateral tibial slide
(thigh technique).*

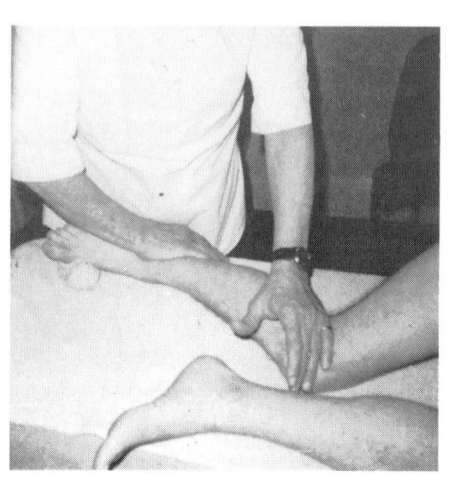

Fibula correction.

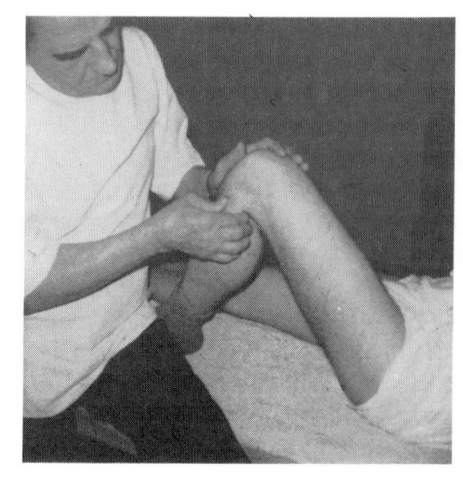

KNEE
Testing fibula movements.

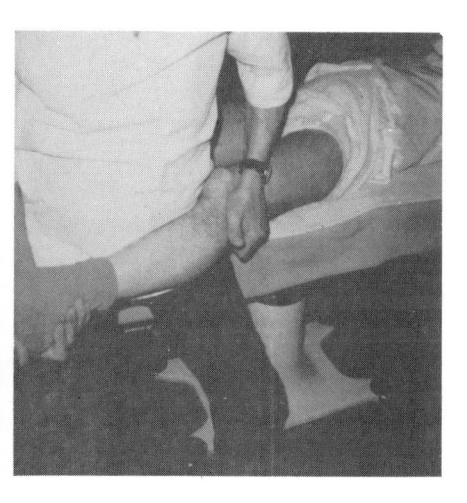

KNEE
Medial slide of tibia correction.

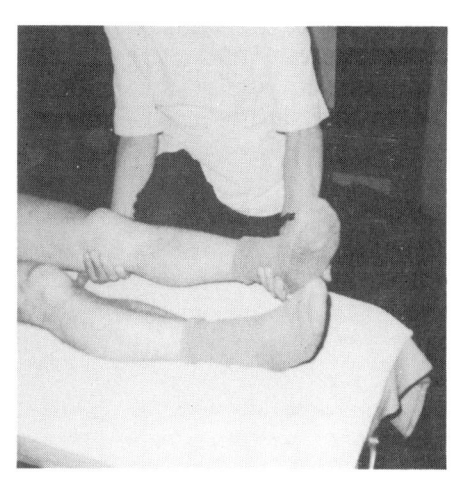

KNEE
Correction lateral slide of tibia.

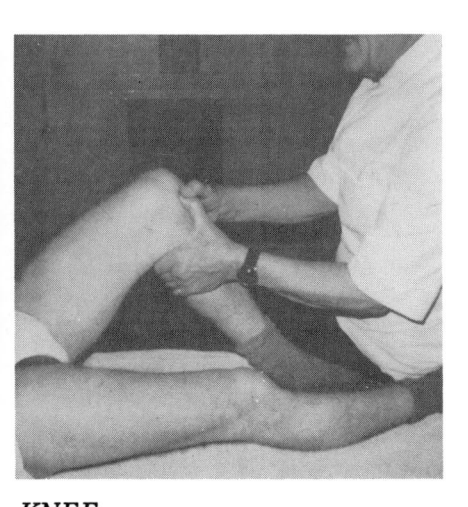

KNEE
Medial cartilage correction. Direct thrust technique.

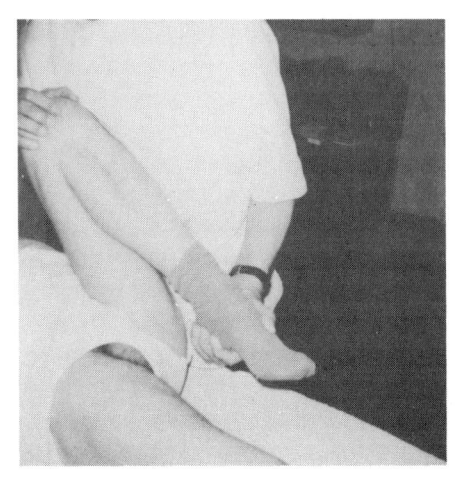

KNEE
Medial cartilage (testing)

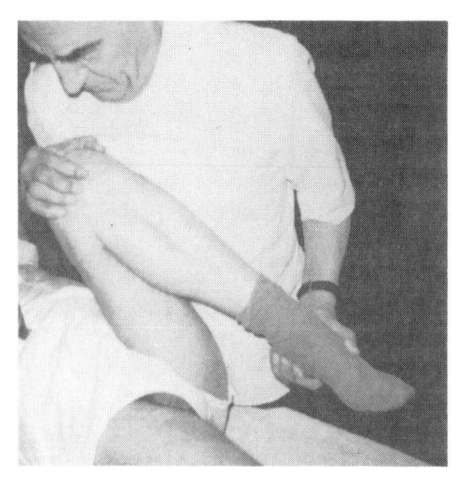

KNEE
Medial cartilage adjustment.

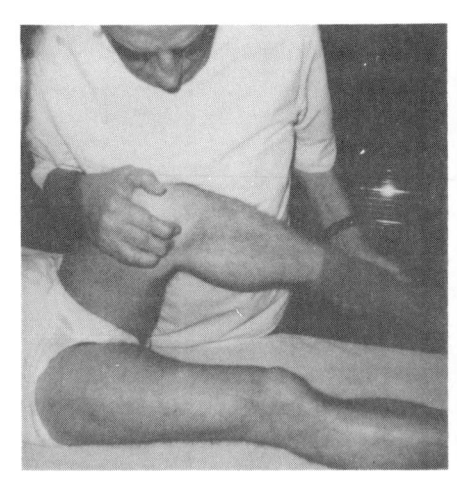

KNEE
Medial cartilage correction. 1

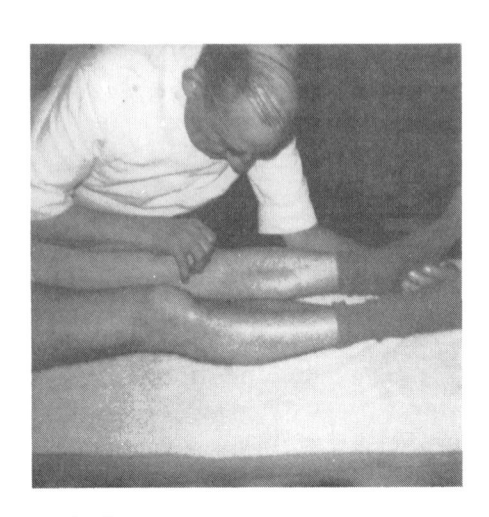

KNEE
Medial cartilage correction. 2

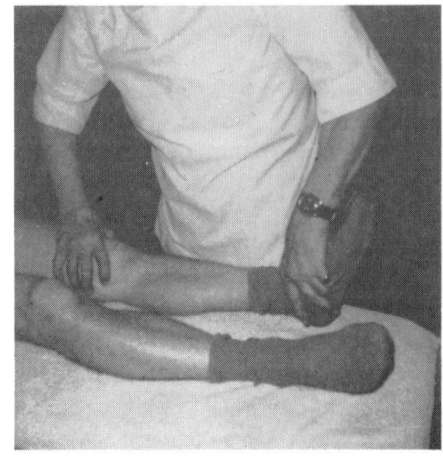

KNEE
*Medial cartilage
Hyper-extension after correction.
3*

THE FOOT

The technique of foot adjustment has probably invited more attention from more practitioners claiming to use manipulation, than any other part of the body. Numerous books have been written by orthodox writers on the foot and with few exceptions, one gains very little from these writers other than orthopaedic alterations in footwear and recent developments in arch supports. In other words, most of the orthodox people rely on crutches for relief, rather than from manipulative adjustment.

Probably no part of the body is more conducive to learning the techniques of osteopathy than the feet, because the majority of these structures are subcutaneous on the dorsum of the foot and allow one an easy means for the study of the art of palpation. One may feel the positon of the bone and the motions of joints more easily than in most other parts of the body. Practise on the feet will assist the student to acquire the art of palpation in the rest of the body.

Many osteopaths have also written a great deal on the foot and its adjustment, notably amongst these are Dr Hiss, Bynam, Styles Jnr and D.L. Clark and of course the famous, or notorious, whichever you like to call him, Dr Post. Now, Dr Post was a very odd man, who managed to sell his foot technique to the American Osteopathic Association, for about 9 or 10,000 dollars. He used to put his thumb or his finger over the bone and hit it with a mallet. I admit it was a rubber mallet, but it was hard rubber! After one or two had broken their knuckles or their fingers at it, it was discarded, but not before they'd paid nearly $10,000!

I agree in the main with the generally accepted idea that most foot troubles are the result of bodily strain. But on the other hand, foot discomforts of varying degrees can be, and often are, due to localised strain either in the foot itself or of the muscles of the lower limb selectively or collectively. You will have probably noticed the preponderance of muscle tissue on the posterior aspect of the lower limb, and it's about this point I wish to speak in relation to the cause and cure of foot conditions. With few exceptions, the aches, pains, wasting atrophy and atonicity, that are common to all foot strains, are found within this posterior group of muscles. There are exceptions of course, where the anterior group appears to be affected. One begins to think of a definite nerve pathology such as injury to the anterior tibial nerve and polio, that show up mostly in the anterior part of the lower limb. Whenever you have to bandage a knee, especially a compression bandage, you should be careful not to have it so low that it covers the anterior tibial nerve, causing pressure on the nerve. That can give you the equivalent to a foot drop, such as you get from strychnine, lead or any other form of poisoning. This results in you stubbing your toe every time you walk along the street, due to the inability of the tibialis anterior and the other anterior muscles to bring the foot up to dorsi-flexion. Therefore while it's true that most of the strains and muscle injuries occur posteriorly the more serious conditions occur anteriorly, the exception being, of course, if you tear the Achilles tendon right through.

The Achilles tendon is rather tough. It's made up of gastrocnemius which is joined into the soleus and they combine to form this powerful tendon Achilles. The plantaris arising from the posterior lateral condyle of the knee joint, is a very small muscle itself, but it has a very, very long strong powerful ligament going down the side of the leg to reinforce the tendon Achilles. I've seen a few, but it's not as common as you think, that an Achilles tendon is torn right through. What happens usually is you get a tearing of a few fibres at the musculo-tendinous junction, which gives rise to pain and weakness. You cannot elevate yourself onto your toes, or walk without heels, and unless you take care of this, you can easily go from that, to, a torn tendon Achilles. When it's really torn through, and you've got a hole there, you can actually feel the hole with your finger. If it's only got a few fibres connecting it to the calcaneous, it's an operation job. It's worthwhile even getting a few cases, and tearing them to watch the operation because it's a beautiful reconstruction job. I've watched a few of these. I always watch my patients being operated on by my orthopaedic surgeon and I've learned quite a lot from it. To see a reconstruction of the Achilles tendon is a thing of beauty, it really is a work of art and they do a very good job.

It would appear that the foot does not appear to be quite balanced by the muscles on the dorsal and plantar aspects. I stress this point because nearly all cases of foot strain show this disparity of muscle in the increase in plantaflexion in the foot in relation to the leg when not weight-bearing. I think here is the reason why we should always endeavour, when adjusting the foot, to commence with the foot in dorsi-flexion. I do not think I can stress this point about dorsi-flexion too much. An examination of the foot would show that any attempt at adjustment of the foot from the position of plantaflexion will only further lock the articulation in question. Now, if there is any 'secret' whatsoever in foot adjustment, this is it. You must never attempt to adjust bones in the foot with the foot in plantaflexion. It you look at any skeleton, you can see that if the foot is in plantaflexion, it locks all the tarsal and metatarsal joints. It locks them, and their plantar aspects are so small, with the exception of the cuboid, that it's very difficult to see how you can palpate accurately through the plantarfascia and the 5 muscle layers of the sole of the foot. It would be difficult to tell whether you're on the medial cuneiform or not.

Now, if you look at the architecture of the foot you might ask yourself, how can a cuneiform or a metatarsal drop? With the exception of the cuboid, it's very difficult for the other bones to drop because if you look at the shape of them they converge. The three metatarsals, the chief ones, converge to a point almost, and the soft tissue from the point of the middle cuneiform to the sole of the foot, is equivalent to almost an inch in depth. This plantafascia and the muscle layers of the foot, are very tricky to get through. They are not made of rice paper; you've got to go through some pretty thick muscles; short thick muscles, which have origins and insertions in all directions, not only vertically, but diagonally. Then you have the peroneii which go down the leg, and underneath the foot and insert in various parts of the first metatarsals and across the metatarsals. There's a very powerful support in the plantar aspect of the foot, which is one of the reasons why you can have the flattest foot in the world and still never have any trouble with it. A flat foot can be a very good foot if it's mobile. You only get pain in a flat foot if something goes wrong and you get torsion of a bone.

There's a film made, a beautiful film of a very flat foot. It's a beautiful thing to see, you see the articulation of the talus, the tibia and fibula and the mechanics of movement is rather lovely. Everybody who sees this film says "that person must be in a lot of pain, the veins show up and the things as flat as a pancake", and yet that person has never had any pain in his foot. I know because it's my foot! A rigid high arch, pes cavas as they call it, is one of the worst types of foot for treatment once they breakdown, and I'd sooner take on 12 cases of flat foot than one case of pes cavas.

I want to stress, when we get on with technique, how we use technique from the dorsi-flexed position. Now, with nearly every technique it is important to try to get to the most neutral position before adjustment. Possibly this goes for the foot, more than any other part of the body, so if you have a cuboid to adjust, you just don't take your thumb and push the foot down. Whatever technique you are using, you take the foot into dorsi-flexion, beyond dorsi-flexion, as high as you can get it. Between that point of high dorsi-flexion and planta-flexion there is a neutral position. You find the neutral position and that is the point and time when you should adjust, otherwise you'll only sprain your thumbs! The foot carried into dorsi-flexion and then slightly released achieves a point of neutrality and therefore gives more complete relaxation of ligaments, muscles and tendons.

Now, Hiss is the man that's usually quoted as the foot expert. He's done very well, and manufactures his own shoes. His first shop was in St Louis, and he himself took over, for a time, the job of chief salesman. He used to wait for people to come in to buy his shoes and before he would let them buy a pair of shoes, he always examined their feet. Of course he found a dropped cuboid in every foot. And so he was always on one knee doing an adjustment of the cuboid. He stresses the value of what he calls his "arch block" technique, (the blocking of the arch which he speaks of is in relation to the navicular and the first metatarsal).

He also relied a lot on his soft tissue work, and on chiropodist's felt and strapping, and yet his book is supposed to be the best book written on osteopathic treatment of the foot. Now, Bynam was a little man; he didn't stand more than 5 feet tall. He came over here and charged us 30 guineas for a course on foot technique many years ago, and some of us were daft enough to take it. But we did learn something from it. He was a man with very powerful short hands, and his technique was all done with thrusts with his thumbs, and cracking of the phalangeal articulations. I have not heard him advocate, except in a general way, any attention to soft tissue being necessary. He didn't consider soft tissue work was necessary to deal with the foot. Clark tends to reverse this approach and apparently pays more attention to soft tissue work and 'remoulding' the foot than the actual adjustment of bones. Styles and Ellis, and Downey and most of the so-called modern foot technicians, appear to think that foot technique is all covered by half a dozen technical methods applied to specific cases of the foot. This is only partly true. There is more to the treatment of the foot than just correction. Many people advocate strapping of the foot, but I don't use these methods any longer as I found them ineffective.

The first thing to do in the examination of the foot is to examine from the pelvis downwards. The knee should receive special attention as any torsion of the tibia or fibula will lead to problems with the talus. An internal or external rotated leg will produce torsion on the talus and have eventual effects on the other tarsal bones. Check the tibio/talar joint. Lesions here must be corrected before moving onto the rest of the foot. In the typical sprained ankle for example, you get an outward rotation of the calcaneous with a forward and inward movement of the talus on the calcaneous. Even in the acute sprained ankle you should try to adjust this condition. You won't hurt the patient if you use the right technique. Apply traction and separation to the calcaneus.

If the tibia is anterior on the talus, which is a common lesion, it interferes with plantar-flexion. This is common in ballet dancers. To reduce this, place one hand over the tibia and the other under the talus. Use a rocking motion of the foot to get mobility into the joint and then thrust the tibia posteriorly while bringing the talus forward. Sometimes this makes a shocking noise and the patient thinks that you have fractured their ankle, but don't worry about that!

Remember, when you adjust a cuboid you will also have a beneficial effect on the navicular because of their articular relationship. You must be on the medial side of the cuboid to reduce a dropped cuboid correctly. To perform the adjustment take the foot into dorsi-flexion and then apply a 'buckling' movement of the foot with your crossed thumbs as the fulcrum. You would remember that trouble with the cuboid always involves the 4th and 5th metatarsals.

What we call the 'figure of eight' technique is a good general treatment for the foot. It opens up the articulations in every direction, but you must change your hands over intermittently if you are to get the full benefits of the technique.

With Hallux Valgus, you must treat the hind-foot first i.e. the relationship of the lower leg to the talus. Having adjusted this area you go on to the mid-foot. The first metatarsal-cuneiform articulation is very important. Only after attending to these areas would you go on to the fore-foot.

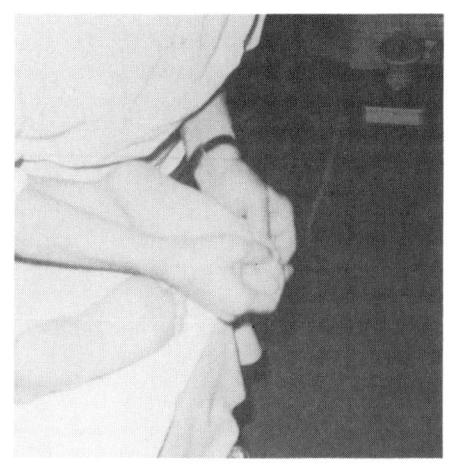

FOOT
Metatarso-phalangeal traction with elevation of metatarsal heads.

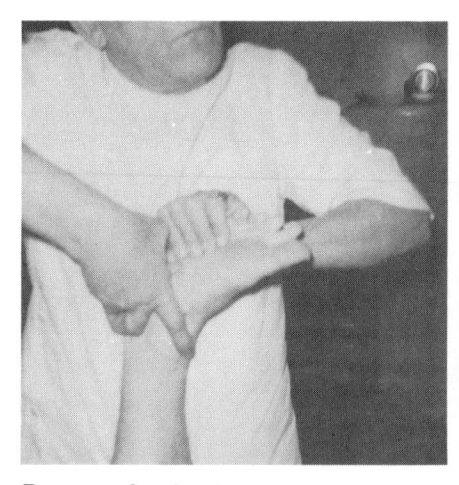

Prone cuboid adjustment.

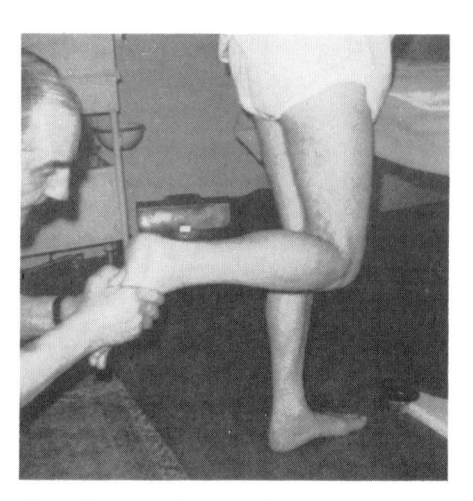

Standing cuboid adjustment.

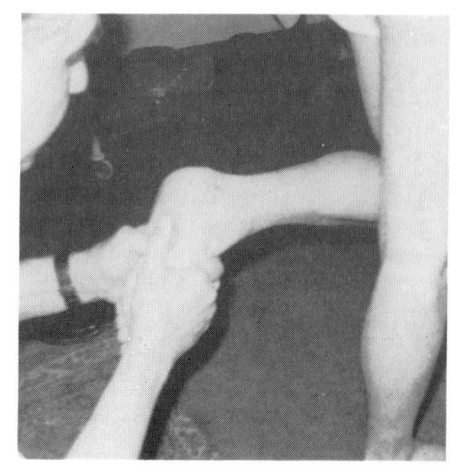

Cuboid adjustment showing crossed thumbs.

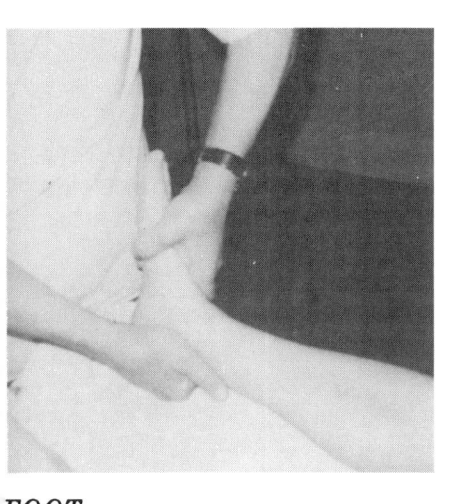

FOOT
Figure eight articulation.

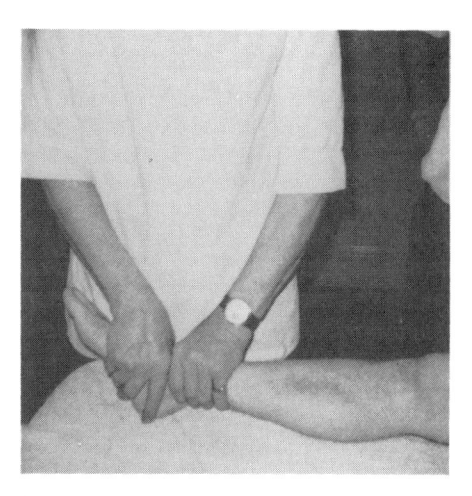

ANKLE
Elevation and depression of the tibia to demonstrate mobility of joint.

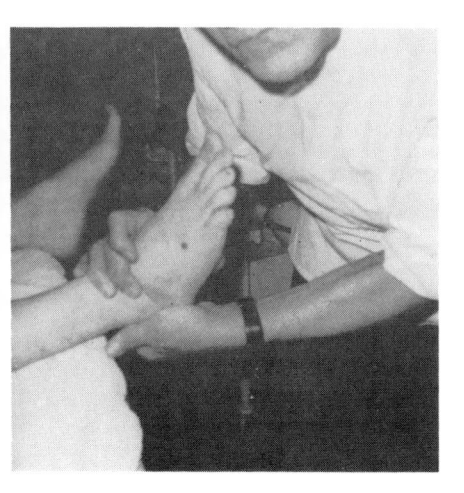

TALO-CALCANEAL
Correction of post lateral lesion.

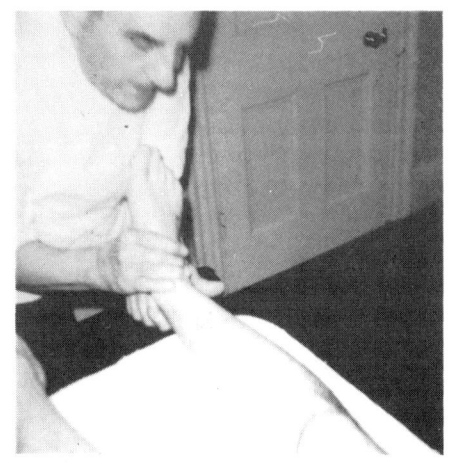

Correction of posterior-lateral lesion.